Copyright © 2012-2015 Fli[

No part of this book may be reproduced in any manner, print, or electronic, without written permission of the copyright holder.

The views expressed herein are those of the authors and do not necessarily reflect the views of your employer, medical director or current protocols.

This publication is intended to provide accurate information regarding the subject matter addressed herein. However, it is published with the understanding that FlightBridgeED, LLC is not authorizing or advising you to engage in unsafe practice or render care above your current state or county protocols. The information contained herein is solely for advanced education for licensed professionals wishing to further their knowledge base. It is not intended for the layperson to provide medical care. It should not supersede each individual's scope of practice or current medical policies and procedures for which the individual is covered under. It is the individuals' responsibility to use their own clinical judgment for decision-making and provide care in a manner consistent with current standards of care. The information in this publication is subject to change at any time without notice based on new research or treatment approaches that are standard in the medical industry. Neither FlightBridgeED, LLC nor the authors of the publication, make any guarantees or warranties concerning the information contained herein. If expert assistance is required, please seek the services of an experienced, competent professional in the relevant field. Accurate indications, adverse reactions, and dosage schedules for drugs may be provided in this text, but it is possible that they may change. Readers are urged to review current package indications and usage guidelines and protocols provided by the manufacturers of the agents mentioned.

Second Edition Printing – April 2015
FlightBridgeED, LLC
Headquarters
520 Old River Rd
Scottsville, KY 42164
Phone + 1 (270) 618-8915
www.flightbridgeed.com

Table of Contents

Preface..2
- Chapter 1) Oxygenation Physiology 3-9
- Chapter 2) Respiratory, Airway & RSI 10-15
- Chapter 3) Dominating Transport Ventilation..........16-23
- Chapter 4) Flight Physiology.....................................24-27
- Chapter 5) Environmental Emergencies....................28-30
- Chapter 6) Hematology & Electrolytes.......................31-35
- Chapter 7) CAMTS Regulations | Operations.............36-39
- Chapter 8) Cardiac Physiology....................................40-46
- Chapter 9) Hemodynamic Monitoring........................47-56
- Chapter 10) IABP Therapy...57-61
- Chapter 11) Endocrine, Renal & Sepsis......................62-70
- Chapter 12) Trauma Management.............................71-80
- Chapter 13) Neurological Emergencies......................81-84
- Chapter 14) Toxicology..85-88
- Chapter 15) OB/GYN Emergencies..............................89-92
- Chapter 16) Neonate & Pediatric Emergencies..........93-97
- Chapter 17) Review Question Rational......................98-180
- Chapter 18) Testing Tips...181

Preface

FlightBridgeED, LLC is a "live" and online educational organization that specializes in providing critical care transition education for the individual wanting to move from ground E.M.S., the Emergency Department, or Intensive Care Unit to the helicopter E.M.S. (HEMS) industry. The project was founded in November 2012 as the product of the combined visions of the FlightBridgeED team. The idea for FlightBridgeED started as a casual conversation and a subsequent formal meeting which resulted in several podcast recordings and an initial deployment of the website. As a community began to develop around the project, the team saw opportunities for improvement and expansion in order to better serve those interested in this very specialized type of education. Listening to YOUR feedback, FlightBridgeED has expanded its vision to develop a complete, multifaceted **"Live" & Online Education System** designed to bridge the gap between ground based healthcare and the air medical industry; A Partnership in Discovery™.

Throughout the past 12 years working in the HEMS industry, there have been many strides made industry wide to bring good quality critical care education to the thousands of Flight Nurses and Paramedics worldwide. Since the inception of FlightBridgeED, we have been driven to bring the best education materials to the industry that meets and exceeds the national standards in critical care.

The goal of this book is to provide the most up to date information based on my experiences, knowledge and current research studies that will make you prepared to take these challenging exams. Whether your preparing to take the CFRN, FP-C, CCP-C or CTRN, we at FlightBridgeED feel like our educational materials will greatly assist you in becoming credentialed in your specific discipline. We feel this separates us from other companies and will make you, the "student", more successful in your testing and career goals. We not only want you to pass these exams, but also want to make you better clinicians and health care providers.

Chapter 1 | Oxygenation Physiology

1) Your patient's current ABGs are:

   pH 7.30, PaCO2 24, PaO2 62, HCO3 16. What is your interpretation?

   a. Uncompensated respiratory acidosis
   b. Compensated metabolic acidosis
   c. Partially compensated metabolic acidosis
   d. Metabolic alkalosis

2) Your patient's current ABGs are:

   pH 7.55, PaCO2 30, PaO2 56, HCO3 25. What is your interpretation?

   a. Uncompensated respiratory alkalosis
   b. Uncompensated respiratory acidosis
   c. Compensated respiratory acidosis
   d. Mixed disturbance

3) Your patient's labs are as follows:

   pH 7.52. Previous pH 7.41 and the K+ was 4.7mEq/L. You would expect the current K+ to be approximately?

   a. 5.3 mEq/L
   b. 5.1 mEq/L
   c. 3.5 mEq/L
   d. 4.1 mEq/L

4) Your patient's initial ABG values are: pH 7.25, PaCO2 51, PaO2 104, HCO3 27, SaO2 97%, EtCO2 54. You have had the patient on your transport ventilator during your one-hour flight. Now your EtCO2 is showing 34. You would anticipate which of the following?

   a. pH 7.43
   b. pH 7.30
   c. pH 7.41
   d. pH 7.40

5) The Bohr effect states?

    a. In the presence of decreased pH or increased acid, your Hgb will release its load of O2 to the tissues
    b. Causes a left shift in the oxyhemoglobin curve
    c. Occurs primarily in the pulmonary capillaries
    d. None of the above

6) Your patient's lab states the current lactate level is 5.3mmol/L. That value suggests?

    a. Metabolic acidosis
    b. Nothing, the value is normal
    c. Aerobic metabolism is occurring
    d. Anaerobic metabolism is occurring / Biomarker for morbidity and mortality

7) When using the "Winters formula" and calculating how PaCO2 affects pH; for every 10mmHg change in CO2, the pH will change by_____ in the opposite direction?

    a. 0.09
    b. 0.06
    c. 0.08
    d. 0.10

8) Your current ABG's are: pH 7.37, PaCO2 58, HCO3 23, Base deficit -2, PaO2 106. What is your current diagnosis?

    a. Metabolic acidosis
    b. Compensated respiratory acidosis
    c. Compensated respiratory alkalosis
    d. Metabolic alkalosis

9) A patient in early shock most likely will suffer from which acid base disorder?

    a. Metabolic acidosis
    b. Respiratory acidosis
    c. Respiratory alkalosis
    d. None of the above

10) When applying rules from the "Winters formula", the flight nurse knows that a change in HCO3- of 10 mEq, will change the pH _____ in the same direction?

   a. 0.10
   b. 0.15
   c. 0.08
   d. 0.06

11) Identify the following ABG's: pH 7.6, PaCO2 23, HCO3 35, PaO2 85.

   a. Respiratory acidosis
   b. Respiratory alkalosis
   c. Metabolic acidosis
   d. Mixed disturbance

12) You have the following ABG readings: pH 7.10, PaCO2 50mmHg, HCO3 24, PaO2 92, EtCO2 50 mmHg, SaO2 92%. You are attempting to manipulate the pH by increasing the patient's MV on the transport ventilator. If you increase the MV to reflect a decrease in EtCO2 from 50mmHg down to 30mmHg, what would your change in pH reflect?

   a. pH = 7.08
   b. pH = 7.26
   c. pH = 7.12
   d. pH = 7.30

13) You are enroute to receive a multi systems trauma patient. You receive ABG results. Which of the following blood gas results would have you preparing to intubate and ventilate the patient?

   a. pH 7.38, PaCO2 44, PO2 8, HCO3 20
   b. pH 7.35, PaCO2 48, PO2 80, HCO3 26
   c. pH 7.03, PaCO2 75, PO2 50, HCO3 16
   d. pH 7.05, PaCO2 15, PO2 158, HCO3 8

14) In a patient suffering from metabolic acidosis, what electrolyte becomes falsely elevated due to the acid base disorder?

   a. Calcium
   b. Chloride
   c. Potassium
   d. Sodium

15) You are transferring a patient from the ICU, post-traumatic injury. The patient has received 6 units of PRBC's. You would anticipate the patient's 2-3 DPG would change and cause the oxyhemoglobin dissociation curve to shift to the _____.

   a. Normal – no change
   b. Right
   c. Up
   d. Left

16) You are transporting a patient from local ICU. You note the patient has consistent NG suctioning and confirm this with the patients referring RN. Based on this, you would expect what acid base disorder?

   a. Respiratory acidosis
   b. Respiratory alkalosis
   c. Metabolic acidosis
   d. Metabolic alkalosis

17) A 70 YO 80kg male who had a recent MI and is now suffering from possible aspiration pneumonia is being transferred for definitive care to a higher-level facility. He is unresponsive and intubated. He has a BP of 110/60, HR 110, R 16/min assisted. He is being mechanically ventilated and has no spontaneous respirations. Dopamine is infusing at 10mcg/kg/min. Current ventilator settings are: AC, Vt 550, f 16, FiO2 0.6. ABG's: pH 7.34, PaCO2 50mmHg, HCO3 19, PaO2 50, SaO2 90%. What would your next treatment priority be?

   a. Increase the FiO2 and f
   b. Wean the Dopamine to 7.5 mcg/kg/min
   c. Continue transporting with no additional interventions
   d. Give a fluid bolus of 250 ml LR

18) Oxygen saturation refers to the % of oxygen that is?

   a. Carried by both plasma and Hgb
   b. Bound to Hgb
   c. Dissolved in the plasma
   d. Also known as oxygen capacity

19) Identify the following ABG:

pH 7.28, PaCO2 20, HCO3 17, PaO2 80, BE-8

a. Compensated respiratory alkalosis
b. Compensated respiratory acidosis
c. Partially compensated metabolic acidosis
d. Uncompensated metabolic alkalosis

20) Acute respiratory failure is defined as?

a. PaO2 < 80 and a PaCO2 > 45
b. PaO2 < 70 and a PaCO2 > 60
c. PaO2 < 60 and a PaCO2 > 50
d. PaO2 < 50 and a PaCO2 > 45

21) A shift to the right on the oxyhemoglobin dissociation curve is caused by?

a. Alkalosis
b. Hypothermia
c. Decreased levels of 2-3 DPG
d. Hyperthermia

22) A shift to the left on the oxyhemoglobin dissociation curve results in impaired dissociation of oxygen from hemoglobin. Which conditions would result in a left shift on the dissociation curve?

a. pH of 7.10
b. PaCO2 of 55 mmHg
c. Decreased levels of 2-3 DPG
d. A temperature of 103.0 F

23) The flight nurse understands that while giving PRBC during massive transfusion, the patient can become more hypoxic at the cellular level. Due to this phenomenon, resuscitation is guided on overall oxygenation status. Why does the patient become more hypoxic at the cellular level?

a. Hyperthermia
b. Hemolytic reaction
c. Decreased levels of 2-3 DPG
d. Decreased calcium levels

24) The flight crew knows that which of the following does not shift the oxyhemoglobin dissociation curve to the left or the right?

a. pH
b. 2,3 DPG Levels
c. Massive transfusion with PRBC's
d. Decreased cardiac output

25) Identify the following formula:

$$CO_2 + H_2O \rightleftharpoons H_2CO_3 \rightleftharpoons HCO_3^- + H^+$$

a. Acid base balance
b. Bicarbonate buffering system
c. Regulation of H+
d. Glycolysis

26) Causes of metabolic alkalosis include all of the following EXCEPT?

a. Decreased levels of K+
b. Decreased levels of Cl-
c. Retention of H+
d. Increased Mg+

27) Your patient is demonstrating an increase in venous oxygen saturation (SvO2) and decreases in oxygen consumption (VO2) and pH. What type of shock do you suspect?

a. Anaphylactic
b. Cardiogenic
c. Hemorrhagic
d. Septic

28) This equation is used to identify what?

[1.34 x Hgb x (SaO2/100)] + 0.003 x PO2

a. Oxygen content in the arteries (Co2)
b. Oxygen uptake by the cells
c. Amount of oxygen bound to Hgb
d. Oxygen uptake by the muscle

29) The flight crew is called to transfer a 58 YOM with acute exacerbation of COPD caused by an underlying pneumonia. The patient has a current temp of 102.1 F. His current V/S are: BP 150/76, HR 108, and RR of 28. His chest x-ray confirmed a left upper lobe pneumonia. His current ABG's are: pH 7.20, PaCO2 68, HCO3 32, PaO2 50. The patient's acidosis and the fever would result in which of the following changes on the oxyhemoglobin dissociation curve?

      a. Right shift with decreased SaO2
      b. Left shift with increased SaO2
      c. Right shift with increased SaO2
      d. A normal curve

30) A 43 YO patient is being transferred to a higher-level facility after being transported by EMS to the local ER. The patient is 2 weeks post discharge from an upper GI bleed. He is currently vomiting bright red blood and has been continuously for the past 12 hours. Current V/S: BP 88/56, HR 128, RR 24. The patient had been given an initial 4 units of PRBCs and the receiving MD has ordered 6 more units. On the flight team's arrival, the patient has received a total of 10 units of PRBCs. The Flight Paramedic knows that the patient will need?

      a. Sodium
      b. Potassium
      c. Heparin
      d. Platelets

31) In the above patient scenario, after the patient has received 10 units of PRBCs, which direction will the oxyhemoglobin dissociation curve move?

      a. Right shift and a decreased SaO2
      b. Left shift and an increased SaO2
      c. Left shift and a decreased SaO2
      d. Right shift and an increased SaO2

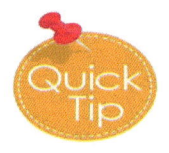

BoHr effect – In the presence of increased acid, the Hgb will lose its affinity for oxygen and will dump it to the tissues. This will cause a high PaO2, and lower

Chapter 2 | Respiratory, Airway & RSI

1) Which of the following does not have bronchodilation effects?

    a. Albuterol
    b. Terbutaline
    c. Decadron
    d. Ketamine

2) Which of the following would you anticipate finding in a COPD patient?

    a. Leukopenia
    b. Polycythemia
    c. Anemia
    d. Thrombocytopenia

3) You perform a needle thoracostomy on a patient with a suspected tension pneumothorax. After re-evaluating your patient, which of the following would indicate that your treatment was NOT successful?

    a. An increase in the MAP from 54 to 76 after the procedure
    b. A sudden rush of air coming from the needle after the procedure
    c. A decrease in the respiratory rate from 36 to 24 after the procedure
    d. A shift of the trachea away from the needle after the procedure

4) You are administering Albuterol to a patient. Which of the following changes would NOT be anticipated with the administration?

    a. Bronchodilation
    b. Tachycardia
    c. Tingling in extremities
    d. Hypertension

5) You are preparing your patient for transfer and the referring RN shows you the patient's current chest x-ray. You note a ground glass appearance on the chest film. Your current vent settings are: Vt 700, f 16, FiO2 .80, Peep 5mmHg. Current ABGs: pH 7.34, PaCO2 38, PaO2 60, HCO3 24. What pulmonary condition do you suspect?

   a. Pneumothorax
   b. ARDS
   c. Cor Pulmonale
   d. Pulmonary edema

6) A 36-year-old man is complaining of increasing dyspnea, nonproductive cough, fever, and increased sweating at night. Upon assessment, you learn that he is HIV positive and has been taking antiretroviral medications for the past 5 years. His current vitals are as follows: BP 118/68, HR 126, RR 36, 92% RA. Based upon your assessment, what would your initial diagnosis be for this patient?

   a. Pneumocystis pneumonia (PCP)
   b. Spontaneous pneumothorax
   c. Cardiomyopathy
   d. Pulmonary emboli

7) Which medication is recommended for sedation of a patient with asthma?

   a. Etomidate
   b. Fentanyl
   c. Versed
   d. Ketamine

8) Non-cardio selective beta-blockers would cause an increased risk of complications in which patients?

   a. Mitral valve prolapse
   b. Grave's disease
   c. Reactive airway disease
   d. 2-day post CABG

9) A 70-year-old female is in acute respiratory distress with a diagnosis of pulmonary embolism. Her BP is 90/60, HR 110, RR 40/min. You know that a pulmonary embolus _____?

   a. Causes hypoventilation
   b. Decreases the amount of inspired oxygen
   c. Increases alveolar dead space
   d. Increases the intrapulmonary shunt

10) Which of the following conditions would put a patient at the LEAST amount of risk for acute respiratory distress syndrome (ARDS)?

   a. Myocardial infarction
   b. Sepsis
   c. Inhalation of smoke
   d. Chest injury

11) You are transporting a patient who recently underwent a thoracotomy. You notice the water in the water-seal chamber of his pleural tube falls during inspiration and rises during expiration. This indicates what?

   a. Tension pneumothorax
   b. Normal finding
   c. The tube not draining appropriately
   d. The tube not in the pleural space

12) What is your priority when treating respiratory acidosis?

   a. Improve oxygenation by placing the patient on a NRB
   b. Administer sodium bicarbonate to buffer the acid
   c. Improve alveolar ventilation by reversing the cause of hypoventilation
   d. Administer an anxiolytic to decrease anxiety

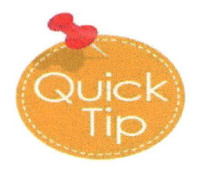

Quick Tip

When performing pre-oxygenation during RSI, use passive oxygenation on spontaneous breathing patients via a nasal cannula @ 15 L/min and a NRB mask @ 15 L/min. Leave the NC in place throughout the entire procedure!!

Eric Bauer, BS, FP-C, CCP-C
Ashley Bauer, MSN, APRN, FNP-C, CEN

13) You are transferring a patient who recently underwent a left lower lobectomy due to lung cancer. He is a 50-pack/year smoker. He is currently on a ventilator with positive pressure ventilation.
When auscultating his lung sounds you notice diminished breath sounds in the right posterior lobe. What do you suspect is the cause of this?

   a. Developing pneumonia
   b. Atelectasis
   c. This is a normal finding
   d. Tension pneumothorax

14) Which of the following can be associated with a poor prognosis in a patient with severe acute respiratory syndrome?

   a. Fever > 103.0 F
   b. Significant leukocytosis
   c. Significant elevated lactate
   d. Increased CO2

15) Oxygen delivery (DO2) is a product of what?

   a. PaO2, MAP, SvO2
   b. SaO2, Hgb, CO
   c. PaO2, Hgb, MAP
   d. SvO2, CI, SaO2

16) You are called to transport a 42-year-old female who is in respiratory distress. She is anxious appearing and diaphoretic. You are told that she has a pulmonary embolus. Her current vitals are: BP 94/62, HR 120, RR 38. You auscultate crackles throughout. You place her on your monitor and note atrial fibrillation. You ask if ABGs have currently been obtained and the transferring RN goes to check. You would anticipate which of the following findings on her ABGs?

   a. Decreased pH, increased PaCO2, normal PaO2
   b. Decreased pH, increased PaCO2, decreased PaO2
   c. Increased pH, decreased PaCO2, decreased PaO2
   d. Increased pH, decreased PaCO2, normal PaO2

17) You have responded to a fire in a building with 5 victims. You notice that a large portion of the synthetic carpet has been burned in the room where you are treating the patients. The patients are exhibiting increasing signs of respiratory distress and coughing after high flow O2 has been applied. What may be causing the patients S/S?

    a. Cyanide
    b. Ammonia
    c. Carbon dioxide
    d. Hydrocarbon

18) You are in-flight with a 70 YOM, cardiac patient, on 6 L/min by NC. You are at 5,000 ft and the patient is becoming hypoxic. What is your initial intervention for this patient?

    a. Decrease cabin pressure
    b. Increase oxygen delivery to the patient
    c. RSI and intubate the patient
    d. Administer a fluid bolus to increase CO

19) COPD patients will commonly suffer from which of the following secondary processes?

    a. Erythrocytopenia
    b. Polycythemia
    c. Thrombocytopenia
    d. Leukocytopenia

20) When evaluating a patient is acute respiratory deterioration; identify the most common finding?

    a. Epistaxis
    b. PaO2 > 100 mmHg
    c. PaCO2 > 50 mmHg
    d. Pulmonary fibrosis

21) You are transporting a 30 YO patient who was involved in a MVC. He has a closed femur fracture with a history of drinking and driving. Which problems may occur in flight?

    a. Histotoxic, hypemic
    b. Hypoxic, stagnant
    c. Stagnant, hypemic
    d. Hypoxic, hypemic

22) When pre-oxygenating your RSI patient, you know the strategy for doing so is?

   a. Displacing the CO2
   b. Causing Nitrogen washout
   c. Improving shunt
   d. All of the above

23) The proper depth of an 8.0 ETT would be?

   a. 21 cm
   b. 23 cm
   c. 20 cm
   d. 24 cm

24) The most common cause of anaphylactic reaction seen from provider administered medicaitons would come from which of the following?

   a. Latex
   b. Morphine
   c. PCN
   d. Neuromuscular blocking agents

25) The purpose for using an opioid like Fentanyl prior to performing RSI and intubation is to?

   a. Improve relaxation for the patient
   b. Improve hemodynamic status
   c. Improve sedation
   d. Blunt the sympathetic response associated with laryngoscope stimulation

26) You are preparing to intubate a patient who has sustained burns over 50% BSA, including airway burns. Prior to administering succinylcholine, it is important to establish the time of injury, because the use of this agent in patients with burns more than 12 hours old can cause serious?

   a. Hyperkalemia
   b. Hypercalcemia
   c. Hypernatremia
   d. Hyponatremia

Chapter 3 | Dominating Transport Ventilation

1) You respond to a small tertiary hospital for a transfer out of the ICU. Initial report from RN is a patient with chronic COPD problems that was intubated yesterday. Current vent settings: patient is on PCV with a PEEP of 15 cm H20, Pinsp of 30, which is providing you with a Vte of 400 mL, FiO2 at 1.0, RR of 32, SaO2 of 88%, PIP 30, Pplat 26. Current ABG results that were just drawn prior to your arrival show a pH of 7.12, PaCO2 88, PaO2 85, and HCO3 26.

RN also says that ABGs as of one-hour ago showed pH of 7.25, PaCO2 60 and PaO2 80.

RN advises you that they are unsure why the patient's ABG results are worse and they are now only getting a Vte of 260 mL based on the same Pinsp of 30.

Patient Scenario #1 Questions
- Obstructive or injury approach?
- Do you want protection with Vt or RR?
- Why are the ABG results worse?
- What is causing the decrease in Vt and poor ventilation?
- What two ways can you use to identify the problem?
- How can we tell what the patient's auto-PEEP is?
- What changes to the current ventilator settings would benefit this patient?

2) You are dispatched for a scene flight with a 6 yo male ejected approx. 10'. Patient is found lying supine on LSB with full c-spine precautions in place in back of ambulance. Patient has a GCS of 8 on your primary assessment. BS are equal with no adventitious sounds heard. Patient with obvious head trauma with a right blown pupil @ 5mm, along with a rigid, distended abdomen and bilateral femur fx's.

You and your partner decide to perform RSI with successful intubation with a 5.5 ETT. You have a good EtCO2 waveform present @ 38 mmHg and bilateral BS are present. You transfer the patient to the helicopter and are enroute to the closest pediatric Level 1 trauma center, which is a 40-minute flight.

You attach your patient to the transport ventilator and place on pressure control ventilation. You check an initial plateau pressure and get 25 cm H20. Approx. 10 minutes later you notice a sharp spike in your EtCO2 and have a reading of 71mmHg. You recheck the plateau pressure and get 34 cm H20. You reassess the vent circuit and evaluate compliance with your BVM, which proves good. All V/S remain unchanged.

V/S – BP 128/72, Pulse 130, SaO2 98% EtCO2 71mmhg, Pplat 35 cm H20

Patient Scenario #2 cont.

- Why is there a sharp spike in EtCO2?
- What is causing the plateau pressure to increase?
- What mode of protection – Obstructive or Injury?
- Tidal Volume or RR for protection?
- What mode of ventilation is appropriate for this patient?
- How can we correct the sudden spike in EtCO2 and Plateau pressure?
- Why is this happening?
- How do kids compensate?
- Why are v/s staying in the normal range?
- What other mode of ventilation can we use?

3) Your patient is demonstrating a sudden elevated PIP with a normal Pplat. The most likely cause is?

    a. Asthma
    b. ARDS
    c. Pulmonary edema
    d. Tension pneumothorax

4) Look at the ventilator settings and ABGs below and make the necessary ventilator changes.

- pH 7.41, PaCO2 40, HCO3 24, PaO2 56; 70Kg male
- AC – volume, Vt 740, f 16, FiO2 .50, I:E 1:2, PIP 42, Pplat 40, PEEP 3

5) Look at the ventilator settings and ABG's below and make the necessary ventilator changes.

- pH 6.90, PaCO2 20, HCO3 15, PaO2 85, 90 kg male
- SIMV, Vt 600, f 16 +18, FiO2 1.0, I:E 1:2, PIP 24, Pplat 18, PEEP 5. Labs: Na+ 138, Cl- 102, K+ 2.1, Glu 581
- Patient was intubated for suspected DKA. Identify potential problems/treatment considerations.

6) Look at the ventilator settings and ABGs below and make the necessary ventilator changes.

- pH 7.20, PaCO2 60, HCO3 22, PaO2 80, 100kg male
- SIMV, Vt 600, f 16, FiO2 1.0, I:E 1:2, PIP 40, Pplat 35, PEEP 5
- Patient was intubated in flight due to massive neural trauma. Patient had associated chest trauma and significant mechanism. Identify potential problems/treatment considerations.
- What is the problem? What's your immediate plan?

7) The main disadvantage of pressure-limited ventilation is?

    a. High FiO2 is required for adequate oxygenation
    b. PEEP cannot be used due to the potential for barotrauma
    c. You do not have a guaranteed MV; higher risk for hypoventilation
    d. Decelerating flow patterns cause poor oxygenation

8) You're flying a 40-year old male patient with a diagnosis of ARDS secondary to acute pancreatitis from chronic alcohol abuse. He is currently being mechanically ventilated on SIMV volume with a PEEP of 20 and he is receiving nitric oxide by inhalation. The nitric oxide needs to be monitored closely for which of the following?

    a. CO
    b. Hemodynamic insufficiency
    c. Hemoglobin levels
    d. Methemoglobinemia

9) When checking for a Pplat. The flight paramedic knows that any pressure above_____ cause VLI and possible barotrauma?

    a. > 50 mmHg
    b. > 30 mmHg
    c. > 40 mmHg
    d. > 20 mmHg

10) Synchronized Intermittent Mandatory Ventilation (SIMV) is described as:

   a. Ventilator delivers breaths at a preset interval with spontaneous breathing allowed between ventilator-administered breaths
   b. Breaths are delivered at preset intervals, regardless of the patient's effort
   c. Ventilator delivers preset breaths in coordination with the respiratory effort of the patient. Spontaneous breathing is allowed between breaths.
   d. None of the above

11) There are two common types of ventilators used in the transport setting, volume cycled and pressure cycled ventilators. When using a pressure-cycled ventilator, the flight paramedic knows?

   a. The ventilator triggers until a preset pressure limit is reached.
   b. Pressure cycled ventilators are preferred with ARDS patients.
   c. The ventilator triggers until a preset volume is reached.
   d. The ventilator delivers a consistent Vt while adhering to pressure limits.

12) In Volume Control ventilation, it is most appropriate to monitor?

   a. PEEP
   b. PIP and Vt
   c. PIP, P$_{plat}$ & static compliance
   d. Minute ventilation

13) Upon your arrival at the referring hospital, you find a 80kg, 25 year-old patient with severe metabolic acidosis who is being intubated, sedated, and paralyzed with long acting medications immediately post-ETT verification. The referring MD transitions care to the flight team. What would be the most appropriate vent setting for this patient?

   a. AC 26, 720 Vt, 100% FiO2, +5 PEEP
   b. AC 12, 720 Vt, 100% FiO2, +5 PEEP
   c. SIMV 32, 400 Vt, 100% FiO2, +5 PEEP
   d. SIMV 16, 600 Vt, 100% FiO2, +5 PEEP

14) You are transporting a ventilated patient who weighs 80kg with Sa02 89%. The patient is chemically paralyzed with diminished lung sounds bilaterally in the lower lobes. Your settings are SIMV volume, RR 14, Vt 450 FiO2 80%, PEEP 4. Which MOST appropriate setting would help increase the patient's SaO2?

   a. Increased I:E ratio
   b. PEEP
   c. Vt
   d. RR

15) Your patient is demonstrating a sudden increase in PIP, however you notice a normal Pplat. The most likely cause would be?

   a. ARDS
   b. COPD/Asthma
   c. Acute ACS
   d. Tension pneumothorax

16) When calculating alveolar minute ventilation you must account for dead space. You do this by subtracting the dead space calculation from current minute ventilation. Dead space is calculated by using which formula?

   a. 50% of Vt or approximately 4mL/kg
   b. 20% of Vt or approximately 1mL/kg
   c. 33% of Vt or approximately 1mL/IBW
   d. 7.5% of Vt or approximately 130mL

17) You are transporting a 56-year-old patient weighing 65 kg. He recently underwent surgery and currently has the following ABG's and is on the following ventilator settings: pH 7.42, PaCO2 38, PaO2 52, HCO3 25. Current vent settings: SIMV Vt 600, f 12, PEEP 5, FiO2 0.6. What adjustment to the current ventilator settings should be made?
   a. Increase FiO2
   b. Increase PEEP
   c. Increase Vt
   d. Increase f

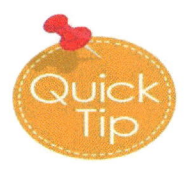

Pplat pressures should never exceed 30 cm H2O. This is a reflection of alveolar health.

18) You are transporting a 30 year-old patient, involved in a MVC, from an outlying facility. The 70kg patient is on a ventilator with an FiO2 1.0, Vt 500, f 16, PIP 22, Pplat 29, PEEP 5. The ABG results are: pH 7.01, PaCO2 70, HCO3 14, PaO2 280, base deficit of -8. What is your ABG interpretation?

   a. Metabolic acidosis with a mixed disturbance
   b. Respiratory acidosis
   c. Compensated respiratory acidosis
   d. Respiratory alkalosis

19) The flight paramedic knows that the pressure regulated volume control (PRVC) mode of ventilation uses a combination of volume and pressure. How does this mode of ventilation accomplish this?

   a. Volume targeted
   b. Pressure targeted
   c. Volume targeted, pressure driven
   d. Pressure targeted, volume driven

20) A 65 year-old-female with a history of CHF presents to the emergency room with increased work of breathing and non-compliance with her medication. The patient stated that she has not taken her medication for two days. She is sitting up on the gurney, currently on a non-rebreather mask @ 15L/min with an SaO2 of 87% and is talking in one word sentences. She has had 3 albuterol treatments and given 40mg of Lasix. On exam, the patient's weight is 120 kg and she is 5'2", she has rales and rhonchi throughout in both inspiratory and expiratory phases. No further labs are available. What mechanical ventilation mode would she benefit from?

   a. Continue current treatment with the non-rebreather mask
   b. Intubate and place on mechanical ventilation via AC mode
   c. Provide 2-phase pharmacological intervention
   d. Place on Non-Invasive Positive Pressure Ventilation

21) You have a 20-year-old asthmatic patient that is intubated for inspiratory failure. Which is the MOST appropriate I:E ratio setting?

   a. 1:2
   b. 1:1
   c. 3:1
   d. 1:4

22) You are called to the scene of an overturned tractor-trailer accident. You are presented with the driver, a 28 year old male who self-extricated himself and was ambulatory at the scene. He is immobilized and has obvious difficulty breathing. Assessment reveals circumoral cyanosis, diminished breath sounds throughout, and shallow chest expansion. SaO2 is 89% on a non-rebreather face-mask. Due to the patient's poor respiratory status, you and your partner have performed RSI, manually ventilated with 100% O2, continue fluid resuscitation, finish securing him to a long board and initiate transport to the closet level 1 trauma center. The patient is placed on a mechanical ventilator for the 40-minute flight. After about 10 minutes, you note increased PIP, worsening chest expansion, and decreasing pulse-oximetry. The most appropriate action is to:

    a. D/C ventilator and manually ventilate the patient, confirm EtCO2 waveform
    b. Increase FiO2 and PEEP
    c. Change to Pressure control ventilation
    d. Check the P$_{plat}$ and if > 30 mmHg perform immediate chest decompression

23) In volume control ventilation, it is most appropriate to monitor?

    a. PIP and inspiratory Vt
    b. Minute ventilation
    c. P$_{plat}$, PIP and static compliance
    d. Vte, and I:E ratio

24) When applying Pressure Support (PS) in a patient on SIMV, what is the stopping point for allowing the patient to take a spontaneous breath.

    a. Spontaneous breaths shouldn't exceed 25% of controlled set Vt
    b. Spontaneous breaths shouldn't exceed 33% of controlled set Vt
    c. Spontaneous breaths shouldn't exceed 50% of controlled set Vt
    d. Spontaneous breaths shouldn't exceed 75% of controlled set Vt

25) When applying Pressure Control Ventilation (PCV), what two parameters do you identify to set your initial inspiratory pressure (Pinsp)?

    a. PS + PIP
    b. PIP + Pplat
    c. PIP + PEEP
    d. Pplat + PS

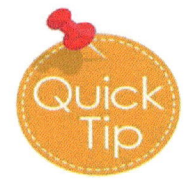

Quick Tip

Maintaining a lower Vt and higher f is essential in protecting the patient from further harm. 6-8 mL/kg is standard. 4-6mL/kg of ideal body weight is standard for protective lung strategy (ARDS, VLI).

In addition, using the proper amount of minute ventilation (VE) is important. Using the formula: 120mL/kg/min will allow you to maintain eucapnia and provide enough VE to overcome the dead space found in the ETT and ventilator circuit.

Chapter 4 | Flight Physiology

1) You are flying at 45,000 ft MSL and you experience an explosive decompression. How much time do you have to apply an O2 source before you experience unconsciousness?

    a. 30 sec
    b. 3-5 sec
    c. 45 sec
    d. 2 mins

2) You would most likely experience barotitis media during which phase of flight?

    a. Level Flight
    b. Ascent
    c. Descent
    d. None of the above

3) Gay Lussac's law states that as you increase the temperature of a gas you would expect?

    a. An increase in pressure
    b. An increase in volume
    c. An increase in gas solubility
    d. A decrease in pressure

4) Barodentalgia will most likely be exacerbated by?

    a. Turbulent flight
    b. Level flight
    c. Ascent
    d. Descent

5) Dalton's law demonstrates that the concentration of O2 at 43,000 ft MSL is 21%. If the barometric pressure @ 43,000 ft MSL is 162 torr, what would your partial pressure of oxygen be at that altitude?

    a. 22 torr
    b. 14 torr
    c. 45 torr
    d. 34 torr

6) You are scuba diving in a local lake and descend to 99 ft below the surface. At this point in the descent you are experiencing how many atmospheres?

   a. 1 ATM
   b. 3 ATM
   c. 4 ATM
   d. 2 ATM

7) When administering high concentrations of oxygen to alleviate hypoxic hypoxia, you are altering which component of which gas law?

   a. Partial Pressure; Boyle's Law
   b. Partial Pressure; Charles's Law
   c. Solubility; Henry's Law
   d. Solubility; Graham's Law

8) You are flying at 35,000 ft MSL and you experience a rapid decompression. How much time do you have before you experience unconsciousness?

   a. 2 min
   b. 30 sec
   c. 3-5 min
   d. 15 sec

9) An expanding ETT in flight is an indication of what gas law?

   a. Henry's law
   b. Dalton's law
   c. Charles' law
   d. Boyle's law

10) Your IABP begins to purge during ascent. The triggering mechanism for this function was initiated as a result of which gas law?

   a. Boyle's law
   b. Gay-Lussac's law
   c. Charles' law
   d. Henry's law

11) Which statement best describes Henry's law?

   a. The sum of the partial pressures is equal to total atmospheric pressure
   b. The amount of gas in a solution is proportional to the partial pressure of gas above the solution
   c. The pressure of a gas is directly proportional to its temperature with the volume remaining constant
   d. At a constant temperature, a given volume of gas is inversely proportional to the pressure surrounding the gas

12) A patient suffering from decompression sickness is an example of what gas law?

   a. Boyle's law
   b. Graham's law
   c. Henry's law
   d. Dalton's law

13) Charles' Law is best defined as:

   a. At a constant temperature, the pressure of a gas is inversely proportional to the volume of the gas
   b. The diffusion rate of a gas through a liquid medium is directly related to the solubility of the gas and is inversely proportional to the square root of its gram molecular weight
   c. At a constant pressure, the volume of a gas is very nearly proportional to its absolute temperature
   d. None of the above

14) As the altitude increases for each 1000 ft, the ambient temperatures will _____ an average of _____ Celsius.

   a. Decrease, 2
   b. Increase, 1
   c. Decrease, 4
   d. Increase, 2

15) The flight crew knows that while flying at cruising altitudes, the aspect of Boyle law causes difficulty in controlling the rate of fluid drips. The most appropriate action would be to?

    a. Stop the IV fluids
    b. Place the fluid on a dial-a-flow
    c. Place the IV on a pressure bag
    d. Manually time the fluids with a pressure bag

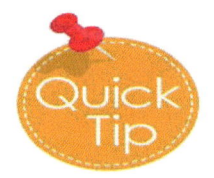

Henry's law can be applied to any patient with an oxygenation problem!

- Increase the concentration
- Increase or add PEEP
- Apply pressure – volume or pressure controlled breaths via the ventilator or BVM.

Chapter 5 | Environmental Emergencies

1) With regard to your hypothermic patient, shivering is limited by?

    a. Cardiac output
    b. Muscle mass
    c. Glycogen stores
    d. Lactic acidosis

2) You are currently transferring a patient in severe hypothermia. Approximately 15 minutes out from the receiving facility your patient goes pulseless and apneic. Current esophageal temp reads 28 degrees C. You know that you should withhold medications until core temperature reaches?

    a. 29 C
    b. 30 C
    c. 32 C
    d. 34 C

3) You are called to transfer a 5-month-old male due to recurrent seizure activity that started today. You note that the baby looks underweight and malnourished. The family says they have no air conditioning. Mother started using tap water for feedings when formula started running low. You administer Valium and control the airway with intubation. How would you treat this patient?

Current labs are:
Na: 120
K: 2.3
Cl: 97
BUN: 22
Cr: 1.1
Glu: 42

pH: 7.24
PaCO2: 58
PaO2: 130
BE: -8
SaO2: 87%
Serum osmolality: 350

What is your interpretation of the labs and current presentation?

4) What is your basic management for warming a hypothermic patient?

   a. Active external, passive external, active internal warming
   b. Passive external, active external, active internal warming
   c. Administer drugs and intubate
   d. Active passive, active internal & passive external warming

5) Which medication below would be the most beneficial for a patient suffering from a heatstroke event?

   a. Solu-medrol
   b. Mannitol
   c. Cimetadine
   d. Adenosine

6) Which of the following statements below is inaccurate regarding heat stroke?

   a. Respiratory alkalosis is a common finding in heat stroke
   b. Oxygen supply exceeds demand
   c. Level of consciousness is decreased
   d. Core temperature can exceed 104 F

7) The hallmark indicator that rhabdomyolosis is occurring in a hyperthermic patient is?

   a. Altered level of consciousness
   b. Increased BUN
   c. Elevated CK levels
   d. Increased troponin levels

8) You are transporting a patient with a history of seizure activity. The patient has been outside fishing in mid-July. Her husband drove her to the closest ER for treatment. Labs reveal: CK 28,000, BUN 68, CR 2.0, and urine is very dark with an output of 20mL over that past 2 hours. She is unresponsive with a BP 100/40, HR 140, RR 28, SaO2 94%. Your diagnosis is:

   a. TCA overdose
   b. Brain tumor
   c. Rhabdomyolosis
   d. ACS event

9) You identify your patient is suffering from malignant hyperthermia. You know this is a result of what?

    a. Massive release of sodium
    b. Massive release of calcium
    c. Massive release of myoglobin
    d. Massive release of potassium

10) The primary treatment in reversing malignant hyperthermia is what medication?

    a. Vecuronium
    b. Fentanyl
    c. Methergine
    d. Dantrolene

11) The flight crew knows that salt-water drowning victims often suffer what type of shift into the pulmonary spaces?

    a. Hyperosmolar
    b. Hypo-osmolar
    c. Surfactant washout
    d. All of the above

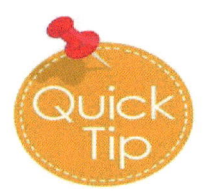

Quick Tip

Depolarizing neuromuscular-blocking agents are the # 1 cause of allergic or anaphylactic reactions, often causing malignant hyperthermia. The medication treatment is Dantrolene Sodium 2 mg/kg.

Chapter 6 | Hematology & Electrolytes

1) Your main focus when treating a patient with DIC is to:

   a. Administer heparin
   b. Administer FFP
   c. Correct the underlying pathology
   d. Replacement of clotting factors

2) You have administered 2 units of PRBCs. Your patient's initial H&H was 6 and 18. You would expect their H&H to increase to:

   a. 10 & 22
   b. 8 & 20
   c. 8 & 24
   d. 9 & 21

3) Which of the following patients would you anticipate being at the highest risk of developing hypernatremia?

   a. 26-year-old male with acute diarrhea and vomiting
   b. 48-year-old female with bacterial pneumonia, fever, and diaphoresis
   c. 73-year-old female with CHF taking loop diuretics
   d. 56-year-old male with CA of the lung and SIADH

4) Your patient is currently receiving a magnesium infusion due to hypomagnesemia (1.2 mEq/L initially). Upon assessment, which finding would alert you to immediately stop the infusion?

   a. An increase in the blood pressure of 15 mmHg
   b. Occasional PVCs on the ECG
   c. Absent patellar reflexes
   d. Diarrhea

5) After reviewing your patient's labs, you notice that their potassium level is 3.1 mEq/L. When looking at their ECG, what would you expect to find?

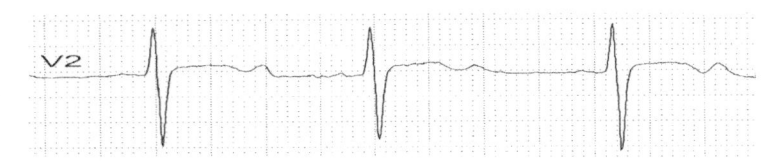

a. ST segment elevation
b. Peaked T waves
c. U waves
d. Increased PR intervals

6) You have a patient with a history of hypoparathyrioidism. They are complaining of numbness and tingling around the mouth and in their toes. You would anticipate which abnormal electrolyte finding?

a. Hyperkalemia
b. Hypocalcemia
c. Hyponatremia
d. Hypermagnesemia

7) Alice is a 72 YO female. Her Hct is 58% an serum Na+ is 156 mEq/L. What is the most likely cause of these findings?

a. Acute renal failure
b. Dehydration
c. Fluid overload
d. Normal finding in the elderly patient

8) You are transporting a patient with a diagnosis of CHF who has been receiving high doses of Lasix. On assessment, you notice generalized muscle weakness, flat neck veins and diminished DTRs. You suspect hyponatremia in this patient. What other assessment findings would help you confirm this diagnosis?

a. Abdominal cramping
b. Dry mucous membranes
c. Oliguria
d. Increased specific gravity of urine

9) DIC is a primary problem with?

   a. Bleeding
   b. Platelet function failure
   c. Clotting
   d. Deactivation of thrombin

10) You are transporting a patient involved in a traumatic resuscitation. They have received 5 units of PRBCs rapidly. What should you be considering in this patient?

   a. Fluid overload
   b. Citrate toxicity
   c. Hemolytic reaction
   d. Methemoglobinemia

11) How would you manage the aforementioned patient in citrate toxicity?

   a. Calcium administration
   b. Benadryl administration
   c. Lasix administration and fluid resuscitation
   d. Methylene blue administration

12) You are called to transport a 26-year-old male who sustained multiple gunshot wounds during a gang-related activity. You are told that the patient required multiple units of PRBCs due to the amount of blood loss from the wounds. You anticipate monitoring the patient's ECG closely for changes indicating what?

   a. Hypernatremia
   b. Hypercalcemia
   c. Hyperkalemia
   d. Hypermagnesemia

13) A 54-year-old male is diagnosed with an acute myocardial infarction. Upon assessment, you note the following:
BP 72/38, HR 118, RR 24, Urine output 30 mL over the past 3 hours CVP 12 mmHg, PAP 32/26 mmHg, PCWP 23 mmHg, CI 1.7 L/min/m2. When evaluating this patient's glomerular filtration rate (GFR), what laboratory value would be best to look at?

    a. Serum creatinine
    b. Urinalysis
    c. BUN
    d. Urine creatinine clearance

14) A 21 year-old man is being transferred to a level 1 ICU after sustaining a venomous snake bite approximately 6 hours ago. He is suffering from the venom and having bleeding from his IV site as well as the initial wound. You notice the referring facility has marked the area of edema and written the time in the area. Which of the following lab values would be suggestive of DIC?

    a. Decreased platelets, increased fibrinogen, normal PT/PTT, normal thrombin time
    b. Decreased platelets, decreased fibrinogen, prolonged PT/PTT, prolonged thrombin time
    c. Increased platelets, increased fibrinogen, normal PT/PTT, normal thrombin time
    d. Increased platelets, decreased fibrinogen, prolonged PT/PTT, prolonged thrombin time

15) The following calculation [Na - (Cl + HCO3) + K] represents?

    a. Strong acids
    b. Corrected anion gap
    c. Cations
    d. Uncorrected anion gap

16) Fluid loss in a dehydrated patient will most critically increase serum levels of which of the following?

    a. Sodium
    b. Calcium
    c. Potassium
    d. Chloride

17) What is the classic sign of hypocalcemia?

    a. Kehr's sign
    b. Grey-Turner's sign
    c. Trousseau's sign
    d. Brudzinski's sign

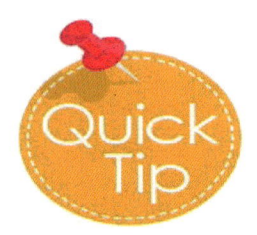

When giving PRBCs, remember your Hgb and Hct will reflect a change upward by 1 and 3 respectively. What does this mean? For every unit of PRBCs, your Hgb will increase by 1 point and your Hct will increase by 3. If you had an H&H of 8 & 20 initially, and you gave one unit of PRBCs, your patient would have a change to a Hgb of 9 and Hct of 23.

In the pediatric population, with severe anemia (hemoglobin <5 g/dL), not secondary to acute hemorrhage, PRBCs should be administered in the amount/kg equal to the laboratory value of the hemoglobin.

Transfuse:

3 mL/kg for hemoglobin 3 g/dL
4 mL/kg for hemoglobin 4 g/dL
5 mL/kg for hemoglobin 5 g/dL

Subsequent transfusions are administered at 10-15 mL/kg to avoid heart failure.

Chapter 7 | C.A.M.T.S Regulations, Operations

1) You have experienced a crash landing. You should rendezvous with your crew?

   a. 6 O'clock
   b. 3 O'clock
   c. 12 O'clock
   d. 9 O'clock

2) The proper shut down procedure for most aeromedical aircraft would be in what priority?

   a. Battery, fuel, oxygen, throttle
   b. Fuel, throttle, battery, rotor brake, oxygen
   c. Throttle, fuel, battery, rotor brake, oxygen
   d. Throttle, battery, fuel, rotor brake, oxygen

3) FAA guidelines state that an aeromedical program may only fly?

   a. IFR in VFR
   b. IFR in VMC
   c. VMC in VFR
   d. VFR in VMC

4) When understanding your aircraft's ELT, the flight crewmember knows:

   a. It may not be activated upon a crash landing
   b. It should activate at 4 G's
   c. It can be manually activated
   d. All of the above

5) During briefing your pilot states that current conditions are "500 and 1". This would mean?

   a. There is a 500' ceiling and a 1 mile visibility
   b. There is a 500 mile visibility and 1 mile ceiling
   c. That he is referring to IFR conditions
   d. None of the above

6) How should your flight suit fit to provide space of insulation per CAMTS standards?

    a. ½"
    b. ¼"
    c. 1"
    d. Skin tight

7) What are the CAMTS VFR Local/Day flying minimums?

    a. 800' ceiling, 2 mile visibility
    b. 500' ceiling, 1 mile visibility
    c. 1000' ceiling, 2 mile visibility
    d. 200' ceiling, ½ mile visibility

8) CAMTS requires how many live intubations upon initial training?

    a. 3
    b. 10
    c. 2
    d. 5

9) According to CAMTS standards, the flight team must respond within how many minutes from the initial time of call to the departure time?

    a. 15 min
    b. 45 min
    c. 30 min
    d. 60 min

10) All of the following are required qualifications for the rotor wing pilot in command EXPECT?

    a. ATP certificate is required
    b. 100 hours must be night-flight time as PIC
    c. 1000 hours must be as PIC in rotorcraft
    d. 2000 hours of rotorcraft time

11) The flight paramedic knows that the ELT is activated with an impact exceeding?

    a. 2 g's
    b. 3 g's
    c. 4 g's
    d. 5 g's

12) You are asked to respond to a scene of a pediatric trauma in an outlying area. The nearest available EMS unit is 45 minutes from the patient. Your pilot is expressing concerns over taking this call due to weather. Who has the final say when turning down a mission?

    a. Pilot
    b. The FAA
    c. Medical director
    d. All crewmembers have equal say

13) A "sterile cockpit" should occur:

    a. During engine starts
    b. On approaches and landings
    c. While flying in air traffic congested areas
    d. All of the above

14) The Flight Team is being transported by ambulance from the helipad to the receiving facility. The local area has seen massive amounts of rain over the past 48 hours. During transport the ambulance comes up to an intersection that is flooded with fast moving water moving over the roadway. What is the best next action the flight team and ambulance crew should take.

    a. Attempt to drive through the flooded roadway
    b. Attempt to identify another route that is safe
    c. Call for back-up
    d. Return to the helipad

FlightBridgeED, LLC

15) The flight team is being transported to a receiving facility via ground ambulance due the facility not having an available helipad. During the 10 mile trip, the ambulance is involved in a minor accident. The Flight Nurse knows that the best place to met up after exiting the ambulance is where?

    a. At the 12 O'clock location
    b. At the 3 O'clock location
    c. On the curb or sidewalk, off the roadway
    d. Remain in the ambulance for safety

16) The flight crew has landed at an LZ of an ATV accident. The ems crew advises you that they will need to bring you into the patient location, which is approximately 1 mile into the woods. Your grab your equipment and your portable radio so as to stay in contact with the pilot and the local EMS dispatch. The flight nurse knows that by using the portable radio, what type of system is being used to communicate with the pilot and dispatch center?

    a. Multiplex system
    b. Simplex system
    c. Duplex system
    d. Digital system

17) You just arrive to work and as you walk in the door your toned for a flight. As you lift from your base airport the pilot calls out on the air-to-air frequency to let other aircraft know of your departure and location in the airspace. What type of radio system is the aircraft using to communicate with the other aircraft?

    a. Multiplex system
    b. Simplex system
    c. Duplex system
    d. Digital system

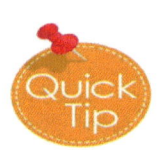

Quick Tip

Condition	Non-Mountainous Local	Cross Country	Mountainous Local	Cross Country
Day	800' – 2 mile	800' – 3 miles	800' – 3 miles	1000' – 3 miles
Night With NVG's	800' – 3 miles	1000' – 3 miles	1000' – 3 miles	1000' – 5 miles
Night Without NVG's	1000' – 3 miles	1000' – 5 miles	1500' – 3 miles	1500' – 5 miles

Chapter 8 | Cardiac Physiology

1) Your patient is exhibiting ST elevation in leads II, III, aVF, V5 & V6. Which coronary artery is occluded?

    a. Right Coronary Artery
    b. Left Anterior Descending
    c. Left Circumflex – LCX
    d. None of the above

2) Your patient is experiencing left ventricular diastolic failure. What would your first line therapy be focused on?

    a. Augmentation of left ventricular clearing
    b. Increasing preload
    c. Decreasing afterload
    d. Decreasing preload

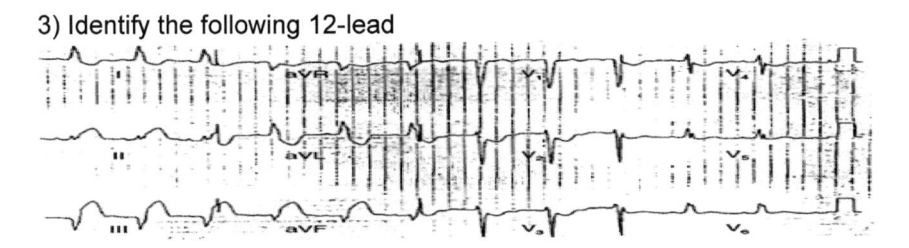

3) Identify the following 12-lead

    e. RBBB
    f. LBBB w/Sgarbossa criteria
    g. Inferior wall MI
    h. Lateral wall MI

4) Your patient has c/o of dyspnea and weakness with the following vitals: HR 112, BP 68/46, RR 30, SaO2 86%, Temp 98.9. The patient is currently on 4 LPM via NC. ECG shows ST elevation with multifocal PVC's. BS reveal bilateral vesicular rales. Exam shows JVD and bronchial wheezing.
Labs: Lactate 5.2, BNP 675, pH 7.13, PaCO2 22, HCO3 16 & PaO2 58
Your most likely diagnosis would be?

    a. ACS - MI
    b. Pulmonary emboli
    c. CHF / Cardiogenic shock
    d. ARDS

FlightBridgeED, LLC

5) Your patient is presenting with ST elevation in leads II, III, AVF. Which treatment below could be hazardous to your patient?

   a. Dopamine
   b. GII/IIIa inhibitors
   c. Nitroglycerin
   d. Heparin

6) You respond to a scene flight for a 60 YOM suffering from chest pain. Upon arrival you note that the patient's BP has dropped after nitroglycerin administration by EMS. The patient is diaphoretic and is complaining of pain @ 10/10. You perform a 12-lead and see ST elevation in leads II, III, aVF. What type of MI do you suspect?

   a. Lateral wall MI
   b. Anterior wall MI
   c. Inferior wall MI
   d. Posterior wall MI

7) Your patient is exhibiting ST elevation in leads II, III, aVF. ST depression is noted in V1-V3. Which of the following may prove hazardous?

   a. Morphine
   b. Isotonic fluids
   c. Heparin
   d. G IIb/IIIa inhibitors

8) When diagnosing a pulmonary embolism on a 12-lead, the flight paramedic knows the diagnostic parameters that he/she should look for are?

   a. Poor R wave progression in the precordial leads
   b. S1, Q3, T3
   c. Lateral wall MI
   d. Positive R wave in aVR

9) The flight paramedic knows that_____ is a drug that has potent alpha effects used to increase SVR in profound vasodilatory redistributive shock states such as sepsis and neurogenic shock.

   a. Dopamine
   b. Esmolol
   c. Nipride
   d. Neo-synephrine

10) The flight paramedic knows what while attempting to diagnose an ACS [acute coronary syndrome] on a 12-lead in conjunction with a LBBB, he/she can use the sgarbossa criteria and knows that to diagnose an MI you would find?

    a. ST segment elevation = or > 1 mm that is concordant with the QRS complex
    b. ST segment elevation = or > 1 mm that is disconcordant with the QRS complex
    c. There is know way to diagnose an MI in conjunction with a LBBB
    d. None of the above

11) Electrical alternans may be caused by?

    a. Pulmonary embolus
    b. Pericardial tamponade/effusion
    c. Tension pneumothorax
    d. Diaphragmatic rupture

12) You are flying a patient via rotor aircraft. Your patient is suffering from an episode secondary to acute cardiovascular disease. You are flying at an altitude of 8,000 feet. This patient is most susceptible to what type of hypoxia?

    a. Stagnant
    b. Hypoxic
    c. Hypemic
    d. Histotoxic

13) Your patient was diagnosed with an AMI 3 days ago and suddenly developed dyspnea and palpitations. He is diaphoretic and anxious appearing. You hear a loud holosystolic murmur at the apex with radiation to the axilla, but do not note an S3 or S4. You auscultate crackles throughout. What do you suspect is this patient's diagnosis?

    a. Right ventricular failure from the AMI
    b. Left ventricular failure from the AMI
    c. Pulmonary embolus
    d. Mitral regurgitation due to papillary muscle rupture

14) Your patient is complaining of a severe headache. Her BP has been ranging from 230/130 mmHg to 210/105 mmHg. She currently has nitroprusside (Nipride) infusing and being titrated. Which of the following medications would you deem most appropriate for this patient?

    a. Lasix to decrease her preload
    b. Labetolol to decrease contractility
    c. Hydralazine to decrease afterload
    d. Nitroglycerin to decrease preload

15) A 68-year-old male is diagnosed with pneumonia with resultant sepsis. His vitals are as follows: T 102.3F, BP 108/68, HR 124, RR 28. He is exhibiting increased confusion as well. What is the initial cardiovascular response to sepsis?

    a. Increased stroke volume
    b. Increased cardiac output
    c. Decreased contractility
    d. Increased ejection fraction

16) What best describes over-sensing?

    a. Failure to sense the patient's QRS complexes
    b. Ventricular failure to pacemaker firing
    c. Pacemaker senses the T wave or other signals and is inhibited
    d. Failure of the pacemaker to respond to atrial impulse sensing with ventricular pacing

17) A 62-year-old female is complaining of chest pain. She has a past medical history of HTN, hypertriglyceridemia, CAD, and DM. Current vitals are: BP 152/90, HR 82, and RR 22. Upon auscultation, you note a split S2 on expiration and single S2 on inspiration. You obtain a 12-lead and note a normal P wave with each QRS complex and PR interval measuring 0.2 seconds. The QRS complexes measure 0.14 seconds and are positive in leads V5 and V6 and negative in V1. What do these findings indicate?

    a. 2nd degree Type 1 AV Block
    b. LBBB
    c. RBBB
    d. Unstable VT

18) Coronary artery perfusion is dependent on?

   a. SVR
   b. Diastolic pressures
   c. Systolic pressures
   d. Afterload

19) A 48-year-old male is complaining of crushing substernal chest pain. You obtain a 12-lead ECG and it shows Mobitz type I, second-degree AV block with ST segment elevation in leads II, III, and aVF. What vessel is most likely involved?

   a. Circumflex coronary artery
   b. Left anterior descending coronary artery
   c. Right coronary artery
   d. Left main coronary artery

20) When treating a patient with a diagnosis of chronic atrial fibrillation, the flight crew knows that _____ medication is most important in decreasing the risk of complications associated with this dysrhythmia.

   a. Warfarin
   b. Propranolol
   c. Cardizem
   d. Digoxin

21) You respond for a transfer of a 58 year-old male with a diagnosis of anterior wall MI. While working on obtaining your initial assessment, the patient becomes tachypneic and short of breath. You listen to lung sounds and hear crackles and auscultate S3 while obtaining heart tones. Based on these findings, what would be your immediate concerns.

   a. Pulmonary edema
   b. Cardiogenic shock
   c. Papillary muscle rupture
   d. Pericarditis

22) You are called to transfer a 67 year-old female patient that was admitted with a diagnosis of anteroseptal MI. On arrival, you note the patient is currently on a NTG drip at 50 mcg/min and dobutamine drip at 10 mcg/kg/min. A pulmonary artery catheter was inserted with a PCWP of 16 mmHg. Current vitals are: BP 128/92, HR 106 and RR of 24. No adventitious breath sounds are noted on auscultation. During your assessment, the patient becomes restless and has cool, pale skin. You decide to recheck vitals and they reveal: BP 102/68, HR 120 and RR of 30 and labored. Breath sounds are still equal but crackles are audible in the bases bilaterally and you note an S3 when auscultating heart sounds. You decide to administer 40mg of Lasix to the patient. You wedge the pulmonary catheter and identify a PCWP now of 8 mmHg with a resultant drop in BP. The most appropriate intervention at this time would be to?

    a. Increase the NTG drip rate
    b. Decrease the dobutamine drip rate
    c. Administer a saline bolus
    d. Initiate a neo-synephrine drip

23) Beta-blockers are contraindicated with?

    a. Narcotic overdoses
    b. Cocaine overdoses
    c. ASA overdoses
    d. TCA overdoses

24) Which type of medication blocks the renin-angiotensin-aldosterone (RAA) system to help with heart failure?

    a. Beta-blocker
    b. Calcium-channel blockers
    c. Angiotensin-converting enzyme (ACE) inhibitors
    d. Thiazide diuretics

25) You are called to transport a patient who underwent a heart transplant approximately 8 hours prior. Upon assessment, you note he is pale, cool, and clammy to the touch. He appears anxious but is alert and awake. You notice JVD and auscultate crackles throughout. Current vitals are: BP 96/56, HR 124, RR 28, O2 @ 97% on 3L via NC. You suspect a decrease in cardiac contractility. Which of the following medications would you anticipate providing for this patient?

    a. Isotonic fluid bolus
    b. Dobutamine
    c. Lasix
    d. FFP

26) Your patient is currently on a magnesium sulfate drip due to refractory ventricular tachycardia after suffering from an AMI. He suddenly becomes hypotensive, experiences respiratory depression, and hyporeflexia. After discontinuing the mag drip, what should you do next?

    a. Administration calcium chloride IV
    b. Increase the drip due to the worsening symptoms
    c. Initiate a dopamine drip
    d. Intubate the patient and continue the current tx.

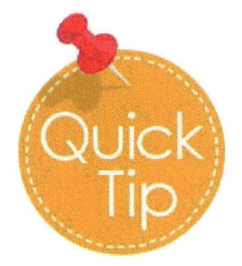

Quick Tip

A LBBB is often associated with ACS and in previous years it was difficult to identify if it was a new or old manifestation. Using Sgarbossa's criteria will assist the clinician in diagnosing an MI in conjunction with a LBBB. Identifying concordant ST segment changes in V1, will give you a probable diagnosis.

Chapter 9 | Cardiac – Advanced Hemodynamics

1) You are requested to a regional medical center to transport a 32 y.o. male that was found unconscious in a lake after a boating accident. The patient was resuscitated by local EMS in the field and flown to the regional facility.

- Intubated with a HR 58, R 12, BP 74/46, Sao2 94%
- Sedated and paralyzed in the field after combativeness
- Ventilator settings AC, TV of 700, FiO2 of 1.0, Rate 10, PEEP at 25
- CVP 0, PA pressures 14/3, Wedge 2, CI 6.4, SVR of 687
  What does this tell you? What is your diagnosis and treatment?

2) **Practice**
- CVP 0
- CI 1.4
- PA S/D 11/5
- PCWP 4
- SVR 1800

- Identify the underlying presentation!

    a. Hypovolemia
    b. Left systolic dysfunction
    c. Neurogenic shock
    d. Sepsis

3) **Practice**
- CVP 16
- CI 1.3
- PA S/D 44/26
- PCWP 27
- SVR 2100

- Identify the underlying presentation!

    a. Hypovolemia
    b. Left systolic dysfunction
    c. Neurogenic shock
    d. Sepsis

4) Practice
- CVP 0
- CI 6.1
- PA S/D 30/14
- PCWP 6
- SVR 400

Identify the underlying presentation!

    a. Hypovolemia
    b. Left systolic dysfunction
    c. Neurogenic shock
    d. Sepsis

5) Practice
- CVP 1
- CI 1.6
- PA S/D 12/8
- PCWP 5
- SVR 300

Identify the underlying presentation!

    a. Hypovolemia
    b. Left systolic dysfunction
    c. Neurogenic shock
    d. Sepsis

6) Practice
You are transferring a patient to a higher level ICU. You identify that the patients PA catheter is exhibiting a large defined waveform with an obvious notch on the left side of the waveform.

The distal tip is most likely located in the?

    a. RA
    b. RV
    c. PA
    d. PCWP

7) Practice
Your patient's PA waveform has suddenly changed to resemble a low amplitude rolling waveform. You know that this indicates?

   a. Withdrawal in the RV
   b. Withdrawal into the RA
   c. Inadvertent advance into wedge position
   d. Normal finding

8) Practice
Identify the following hemodynamic waveform:

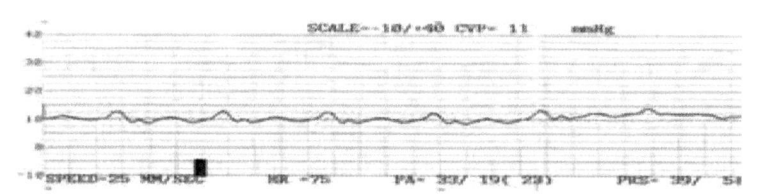

9) Practice
Identify the following hemodynamic waveform:

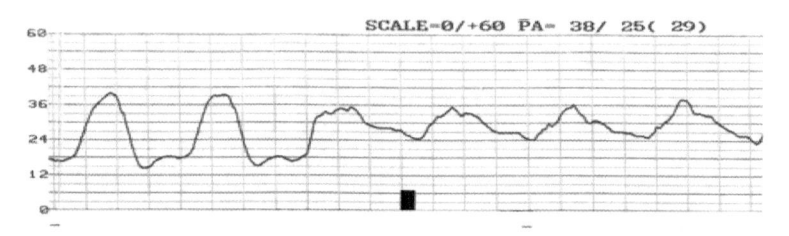

10) Practice
Identify the following hemodynamic waveform:

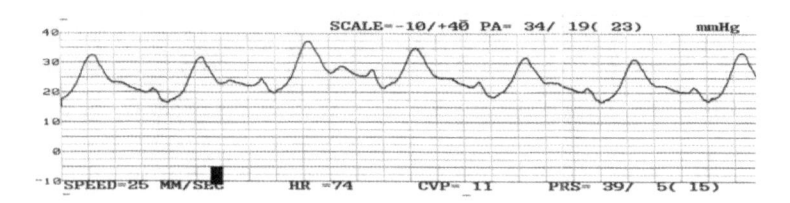

11) Practice
Identify the following hemodynamic waveform:

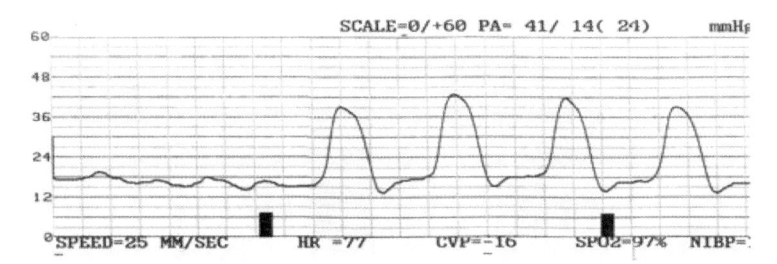

```
                    SCALE=0/+60  PA= 41/ 14( 24)           mmHg
60
48
36
24
12
   SPEED=25 MM/SEC    HR =77    CVP=-16    SPO2=97%  NIBP=
```

12) Pulmonary capillary wedge pressure (PCWP) looks at what?

   a. Afterload of the heart
   b. Right sided preload
   c. Right sided ventricular pressures
   d. Directly reflects left atrial pressure

13) When obtaining a PCWP on your cardiac patient, you note a large V wave on the waveform. After confirming that the PA catheter is correctly placed and the balloon is not ruptured, what condition do you suspect?

   a. Tricuspid valve regurgitation
   b. Pulmonic valve stenosis
   c. Aortic valve stenosis
   d. Mitral valve regurgitation

14) The dicrotic notch on the arterial waveform is reflective of what mechanical event in the heart?

   a. Tricuspid valve closure
   b. Pulmonic valve closure
   c. Mitral valve closure
   d. Aortic valve closure

15) A normal CVP/RAP reading would be?

   a. 6-10 mmHg
   b. 2-6 mmHg
   c. 12-16 mmHg
   d. 22-28 mmHg

FlightBridgeED, LLC

16) You note the following hemodynamic parameters: CVP 2, PCWP 12, CI 1.5, SVR 1800. What is your clinical diagnosis?

   a. Cardiogenic shock
   b. Hypovolemic shock
   c. Neurogenic shock
   d. Sepsis

17) You are transporting a patient from the ICU that is 2 days post trauma. You are packaging her for transport and the referring RN gives you her hemodynamic parameters. They are as follows: CVP 2, PCWP 8, CI 2.2, SVR 400. What is your diagnosis?

   a. Right sided MI
   b. Hypovolemic shock
   c. Neurogenic shock
   d. Cardiogenic shock

18) Which of the following hemodynamic parameters is most indicative of cardiogenic shock?

   a. Systolic BP 80mmHg, CI 1.8L/min, PCWP 30mmHg
   b. Systolic BP 90mmHg, CI 2.2L/min, PCWP 5mmHg
   c. Systolic BP 120mmHg, CI 4L/min, PCWP 12mmHg
   d. Systolic BP 140mmHg, CI 3L/min, PCWP 8mmHg

19) A patient with an extensive anterior wall myocardial infarction has a BP of 88/60, PCWP 8mmHg, and CI 2.0L/min. Which of the following diagnoses best describes this condition?

   a. Ventilation perfusion disorder
   b. Activity intolerance secondary to imbalance between supply and demand
   c. Fluid volume excess secondary to decreased CO
   d. Decreased CO secondary to decreased myocardial contractility.

20) The central line readings obtained in the ICU prior to transport of a patient are as follows: CVP 13, CI 1.4, and a PCWP 18. This could indicate what problem for the patient?

   a. Hypovolemic shock
   b. Septic shock
   c. Cardiogenic shock
   d. Anaphylactic shock

21) You note the following hemodynamic parameters: CVP 2, PCWP 10, CI 1.8, and SVR 400. What is your diagnosis?

   a. Neurogenic shock
   b. Septic shock
   c. Hypovolemic shock
   d. Anaphylactic shock

22) What is the normal SVR measurement?

   a. 200-400 dyne-sec/cm
   b. 400-1000 dyne-sec/cm
   c. 800-1200 dyne-sec/cm
   d. 1200-1800 dyne-sec/cm

23) How is cardiac output determined?

   a. CO=SV X HR
   b. CO=MAP – HR
   c. CO=BP X HR
   d. None of the above

24) What is the formula for determining MAP?

   a. MAP = (HR + DBP) / 2
   b. MAP = [(SBP + (2 x DBP) / 3]
   c. MAP = [SBP +(2 x DBP)/ 2]
   d. None of the above

25) The_____measures filling pressures on the right side of the heart as the tip lies in right atrium.

   a. PCWP
   b. CVP
   c. End left diastolic pressure
   d. RV pressure

26) The flight nurse knows the normal SvO2 (central venous oxygen concentration)?

   a. 70-90%
   b. 50-60%
   c. 30-60%
   d. 60-80%

27) What is the normal range for a PCWP?

a. 4-9 mmHg
b. 6-10 mmHg
c. 8-12 mmHg
d. 12-15 mmHg

28) When attempting to "wedge" a PA catheter, the flight paramedic knows:

a. Fill the balloon with exactly 2 mL
b. Fill the balloon with up to 1.5 mL, but no more
c. Fill the balloon with exactly 2.5 mL, but no more
d. Fill the balloon with 1 mL, but may exceed 2 mL

29) Which of the following pulmonary artery pressures are within normal limits.

a. PAP 34/24, PCWP 12
b. PAP 30/20, PCWP 10
c. PAP 28/18, PCWP 20
d. PAP 24/14, PCWP 12

30) Which of the following hemodynamic parameters would indicate left ventricular failure in a patient with COPD?

a. PAP 25/21, PCWP 13
b. PAP 48/26, PCWP 12
c. PAP 22/12, PCWP 16
d. PAP 48/26, PCWP 20

31) Your patient is a 50-year-old complaining of pain in her chest that is radiating to her (L) arm and up into her jaw. She is alert, diaphoretic, and appears anxious. You note an audible S3 at the apex and crackles throughout the lung bases. Vitals and hemodynamic parameters are as follows: BP: 80/60mmHg, HR 118bpm, CVP 3mmHg, PAP 40/24mmHg, PCWP 20mmHg, CI 3.6L/min, SVR 1340 dynes/sec/cm-5. While utilizing inotropes and vasodilators to maintain optimal PCWP, which of the following parameters would you determine optimal for this patient?

a. PCWP 16, CI 2.5, BP 96/60, urine output 12mL/hr
b. PCWP 18, CI 2.5, BP 100/60, urine output 20mL/hr
c. PCWP 26, CI 1.2, BP 80/50, urine output 10mL/hr
d. PCWP 12, CI 1.9, BP 95/60, urine output 15mL/hr

32) What would most likely cause dyspnea with a normal PCWP, an increase in pulmonary artery diastolic pressure (PAD), an increase in pulmonary vascular resistance (PVR), and an increase in CVP?

   a. Myocardial infarction
   b. Pulmonary embolism
   c. Cardiac tamponade
   d. Right ventricular failure

33) While transferring a patient out of the ICU, the flight nurse notes the patient's current hemodynamic parameters. His current CI is 1.6, CVP 17, PAP 44/22 mmHg, and PCWP 18 with a current BP of 78/60 and HR of 120. These hemodynamic parameters would suggest what diagnosis?

   a. Neurogenic shock
   b. Right ventricular infarction
   c. Septic shock
   d. Cardiogenic shock

34) Normal values for the monitoring of PA pressures are:

   a. 2-6/8-14 mmHg
   b. 20-30/10-15 mmHg
   c. 25-35/20-30 mmHg
   d. 30-35/25-35 mmHg

35) Your patient's peripheral A-line is showing a very sharp waveform with readings that appear exaggerated. This may be due to:

   a. Catheter whip
   b. Over dampening of the pressure system
   c. Kinking of the pressure tubing
   d. Catheter embolus formation

36) Central venous pressure monitors:

   a. Intra-arterial pressure
   b. Pulmonary artery pressure
   c. Right atrial pressure
   d. Femoral venous pressure

37) A common cause of elevated PA pressures is?

   a. Left ventricular failure
   b. Mitral valve stenosis
   c. Mitral valve regurgitation
   d. All of the above

38) The central line reading obtained in the ICU prior to your arrival shows: CVP 13, CI 1.4, and PCWP 18. This could indicate what problem for the patient?

   a. Hypovolemia
   b. Heart failure
   c. Anaphylactic shock
   d. None of the above

39) You notice that your patient has the following waveform and is showing VT on the monitor. Your initial intervention for the patient is to?

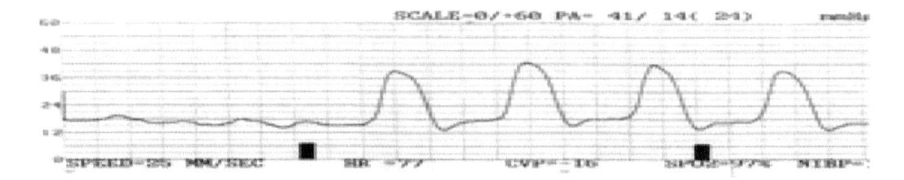

   a. Synchronize cardioversion
   b. Advance the catheter by inflating the balloon
   c. Administer a precordial thump
   d. Pull catheter back into the CVP position

40) The patient's PA catheter is exhibiting a large, well-defined waveform with an obvious "notch" on the left side of the waveform. The distal tip is most likely located in the:

   a. RA
   b. PA
   c. PCWP
   d. RV

41) Your patient has the following parameters: CVP 28, CI 1.2, PA S/D 48/29, PCWP 27 and SVR 1700: What diagnosis could you make?

    a. Right sided MI/Right ventricular infarct
    b. Septic shock
    c. Cardiogenic shock
    d. Pulmonary embolism

42) You respond for an interfacility transfer of an 18 yo male that was transported by EMS secondary to a gunshot wound to the chest. On your initial assessment you find that the patient has distant heart tones, JVD with the head elevated at 45 degrees, and associated hypotension. You suspect the patient is suffering from Beck's triad and a cardiac tamponade. The referring MD has placed a pulmonary artery catheter. Along with a decreased and compromised cardiac output, what would you predict the other hemodynamic numbers would reveal?

    a. Decreased CVP, Increased PCWP
    b. Increased CVP, Increased PCWP
    c. Decreased CVP, Decreased PCWP
    d. Increased CVP, Decreased PCWP

43) When transporting and assessing a patient with a pulmonary catheter, the flight nurse knows that if the PAP is more that 5 mmHg above the PCWP, it signals which abnormal condition is occurring?

    a. High SVR
    b. Pulmonary hypertension
    c. Left ventricular failure
    d. Mitral valve insufficiency

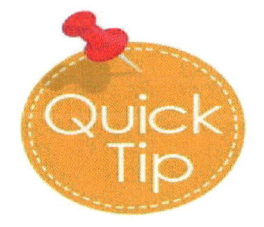

> **Quick Tip**
>
> *Your patient's CVP will guide your care. A high CVP tells you the patient is either fluid overloaded or there's a problem down stream (left side of the heart). A low CVP tells you the patient is preload depleted or they are suffering from a vasogenic or distributive shock!*

Chapter 10 | Cardiac – IABP therapy

1) What is the timing error?

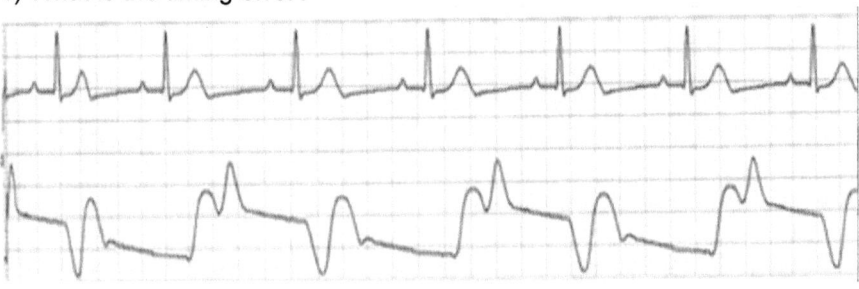

2) What is the timing error?

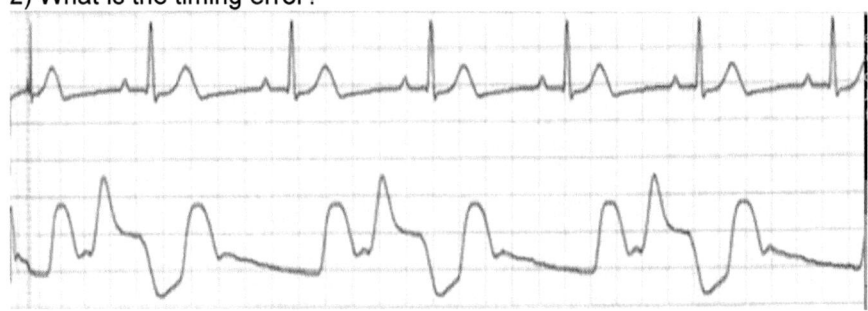

3) What is the timing error?

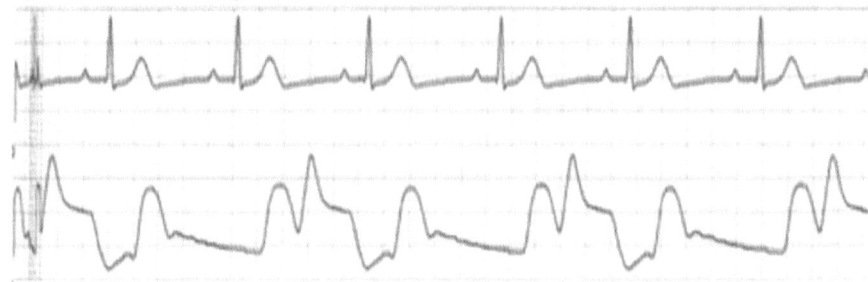

4) What is the timing error?

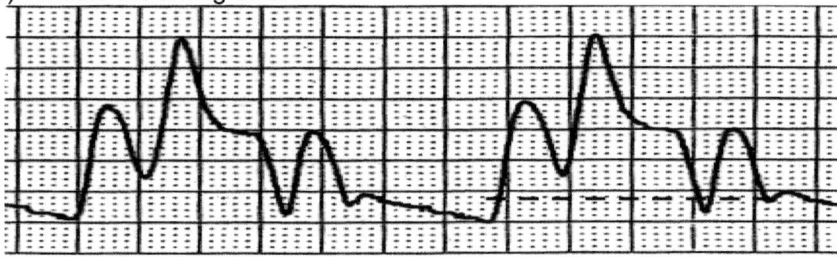

5) What is the primary trigger for the IABP?

    a. A-line
    b. PA cath
    c. ECG
    d. EtCO2 waveform

6) Which timing error is the most harmful?

    a. Early inflation
    b. Late inflation
    c. Late deflation
    d. All of the above

7) During level flight you experience complete power failure of your IABP. What would your most important action be?

    a. Cycle the balloon manually; timing with the ECG
    b. Cycle the balloon manually; timing with the A-Line
    c. Withdrawal the IABP catheter to 10 cm mark
    d. Manually inflate the IABP balloon every 30 min; regardless of timing

8) The balloon has dislodged while treating your IABP patient. Which is the most common site that will be affected.

    a. Right radial
    b. Left radial
    c. Right femoral
    d. Left femoral

FlightBridgeED, LLC

9) What is the most ominous timing error that can occur while transporting a patient on an IABP?

    a. Early deflation
    b. Late deflation
    c. Late inflation
    d. Early deflation

10) During transport, you note rust colored "flakes" in the IABP tubing. This indicates?

    a. Helium tank degradation
    b. IABP failure
    c. Helium oxidation
    d. IABP balloon rupture

11) The secondary trigger used for most IABP operations is the?

    a. A–Line
    b. PA catheter
    c. ECG waveform
    d. CVP waveform

12) Inadvertent migration of the IABP may cause which of the following, EXCEPT:

    a. Loss of renal perfusion
    b. Loss of flow to the carotid vein
    c. Loss of flow to the renal arteries
    d. Loss of flow to the subclavian artery

13) The IABP is indicated in all the following patients EXCEPT:

    a. Cardiogenic shock
    b. Unstable angina
    c. Aortic insufficiency
    d. Weaning from cardiopulmonary bypass

14) You are transporting a patient on an IABP. During transport you notice that the patients urine output has stopped. What is the problem?

    a. Balloon rupture
    b. Renal artery occlusion due to balloon migration
    c. Subclavian artery occlusion due to balloon migration
    d. All of the above

15) The flight paramedic is transporting a patient on an IABP. During transport he/she notices this timing waveform. Identify this waveform:

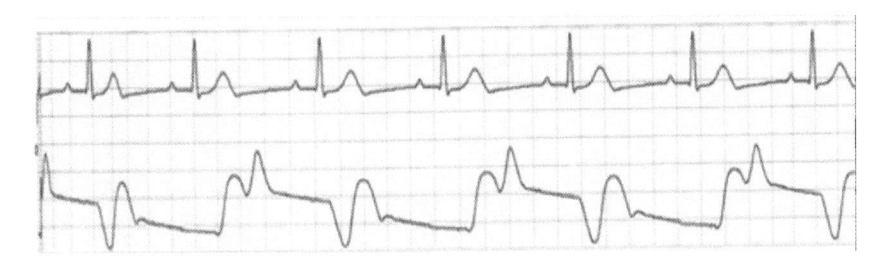

a. Early inflation; early deflation
b. Late inflation; early deflation
c. Late inflation; late deflation
d. Early inflation; late deflation

16) While setting up your IABP, the flight paramedic knows that the standard timing ratio is?

a. 1:1
b. 1:2
c. 1:3
d. None of the above

17) Which of the following pressures is augmented by the IABP inflation?

a. End systolic left ventricular pressure
b. Aortic diastolic pressure
c. Aortic systolic pressure
d. Left ventricular diastolic pressure

18) All IABP systems use helium as the drive gas because of which of the following characteristics?

a. Low density
b. High density
c. High molecular weight
d. All the above

19) While monitoring the arterial line of a patient with an IABP, the balloon should show diastolic augmentation at what part of the arterial waveform?

    a. Dicrotic notch
    b. Systolic phase
    c. Ventricular ejection phase
    d. Anacrotic notch on RV waveform

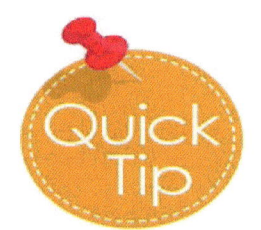

The most harmful timing error while performing IABP therapy is LATE DEFLATION. Late deflation impedes diastolic augmentation and coronary artery perfusion due to the balloon being inflated during the start of the systolic phase. This causes increased afterload, increased myocardial oxygen consumption and poor coronary perfusion. WORST TIMING ERROR!!

Chapter 11 | Endocrine, Renal & Sepsis

1) You are performing an assessment on your patient and you note that your patient "winces" as you are palpating their RUQ. What is the most likely cause of this patient's pain?

    a. Costochondritis
    b. Splenic injury
    c. Gallbladder
    d. Stomach

2) You are dispatched to a scene flight with a man who has fallen approximately 10 feet off a ladder striking his (L) lower rib region on the corner of a patio set. He is complaining of pain in the tip of his (L) shoulder. Which organ are you most concerned about?

    a. Stomach
    b. Spleen
    c. Liver
    d. Lung

3) You are requested to transport a 32-year-old female diagnosed with DKA. She is 5'4" weighing 86 kg. While in the ED, she has been breathing at a rate of 38 and you notice upon assessment that the patient appears fatigued. You make the decision to intubate the patient and request current ABGs. They are as follows: pH 7.01, PaCO2 23, PaO2 280, HCO3 17. She is currently on a NRB at 15LPM. Which of the following plans would best suit this patient initially?

    a. Continue paralysis and sedation after intubation and set vent to: VC, SIMV, rate 12, FiO2 0.6, Vt 870, PEEP 5
    b. Continue paralysis and sedation after intubation and set vent to: VC, AC, rate 12, FiO2 0.7, Vt 600, PEEP 5
    c. Continue sedation after intubation and set vent to: VC, AC, rate 30, FiO2 0.7, Vt 850, PEEP 5
    d. Continue sedation after intubation and set vent to: VC, SIMV, rate 30, FiO2 0.6, Vt 500, PEEP 5

4) You are transporting a 58-year-old male diagnosed with SIADH. What is considered appropriate therapy for you to do while transporting this patient?

    a. Administer an aldosterone substitute such as fludrocortisone (Florinef)
    b. Administer furosemide
    c. Administer vasopressin
    d. Provide aggressive hydration and fluid resuscitation

5) You are transporting a 23-year-old male who has sustained traumatic injuries after being involved in an MVC. He has become hypovolemic and is demonstrating signs of shock. Which of the following would you also anticipate along with this?

    a. Pre-renal failure
    b. Renal failure
    c. Post-renal failure
    d. None of the above

6) You are called to transport a 26-year-old patient in DKA. Which of the following assessment findings would indicate that this patient's DKA is deteriorating?

    a. Urine pH less than 5.8
    b. An increase in bicarb from 22 mEq/L to 25 mEq/L
    c. DTRs decreasing from +2 to +1
    d. Potassium levels decreasing from 6.3 mEq/L to 5.2 mEq/L

7) Which would be the best choice to treat someone with DI?

    a. Aggressive correction of acidosis using bicarbonate administration and respiratory compensation
    b. Aggressive glucose control with insulin
    c. Aggressive fluid management with DDAVP
    d. Aggressive diuresis using diuretics

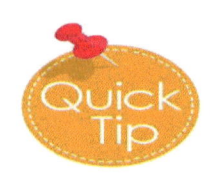

Quick Tip: *Diabetes Insipidus is caused by inadequate or no ADH production or release from the pituitary gland. This disease is secondary to a lack of vasopressin hormone. This causes excessive urination and Na+ concentration buildup. Treatment is targeted around Desmopressin (DDAVP). DDAVP is a synthetic form of vasopressin. It works on the kidneys to help decrease the amount of urine made.*

8) You are transporting a patient with ARDS, exceptionally elevated WBC, elevated bands and a positive Cullen's sign. He also c/o upper abdominal pain. He has a history of alcoholism with frequent nausea and vomiting and has not routinely received any medical care. His CXR is showing infiltrates, patchy and diffuse, in the (L) lower field and elevation of the (L) side of the diaphragm. He describes his pain as constant and severe. What would his diagnosis likely be?

    a. Acute GI perforation and hemorrhage
    b. Acute hepatitis
    c. Acute pancreatitis
    d. Acute appendicitis

9) A 32-year old man presents with fever, hyperglycemia and increasing confusing for the past four hours. HR 146/min, resp 32/min, and BP 82/48 mmHg. Upon assessment you note dry mucous membranes and capillary refill of 4 sec. Current labs are: K+ 3.0 mEq/L, glucose 485 mg/dL and ABGs show a pH of 7.1. Which of the following types of fluids is most appropriate initially for this patient?

    a. LR
    b. 0.9% NS
    c. 0.45% NS
    d. 3% NS

10) Which of the following laboratory findings would you expect to see in a patient with the diagnosis of SIADH?

    a. Hypoglycemia
    b. Dilutional hyponatremia
    c. Hyperkalemia
    d. Dilutional hypercalcemia

11) A 76-year-old male presents with a 4-day history of fever, cough, and (L) sided pleuritic pain. The patient's family states that he has become more lethargic and dizzy with several frequent falls. Vital signs are: WBC 17.2, HR 124, BP 72/38, T 102.0F, R 32/min, O2 82% on RA. His CXR shows a LLL infiltrate. Which of the following best fits this patient?

    a. SIRS
    b. Sepsis
    c. Severe Sepsis
    d. Septic Shock

12) List 6 goals of initial resuscitation of sepsis-induced hypoperfusion to be achieved within the first 6 hours of resuscitation.
   1)
   2)
   3)
   4)
   5)
   6)

13) A 76-year-old woman was recently started on enteral feedings at a long-term care facility. She was transferred to the local ER due to a change in level of consciousness. You were called for a transfer flight and received report. Current labs are: Na+ 150, BUN 80 mg/dL, serum glucose 870 mg/dL, & serum osmolality of 377 mOsm/kg. What is the most likely cause of the serum osmolality being abnormal?

   a. Overhydration
   b. SIADH
   c. Dehydration
   d. Over use of diuretics

14) When treating the septic patient, the goal for initial fluid resuscitation is?

   a. 10mL/kg
   b. 15mlLkg
   c. 20mL/kg
   d. 30mL/kg

15) Which lab finding would be most associated with diabetes insipidus?

   a. Elevated capillary blood glucose
   b. Relative hyperkalemia
   c. Relative hypocalcemia
   d. Urinary hypo-osmolality

16) A key component used in the management of both DKA and HHNK is?

   a. Aggressive fluid resuscitation
   b. Rapid correction of the high glucose
   c. Aggressive correction of the metabolic acidosis
   d. Aggressive correction of the associated hyperkalemia

17) Systemic inflammatory response syndrome (SIRS) can lead to multi-organ dysfunction. Which of the following organs is involved first?

    a. Brain
    b. Liver
    c. Lungs
    d. Heart

18) You are treating a 15-year-old girl who is very lethargic and only responsive to painful stimuli. She has a history of type I diabetes mellitus and has been sick with a virus for the past couple of days. When reviewing her lab results, what would you expect to find?

    a. Hyperglycemia, hypokalemia, acidosis, elevated serum osmolality
    b. Hyperglycemia, hyperkalemia, acidosis, elevated serum osmolality
    c. Hyperglycemia, hypokalemia, alkalosis, elevated serum osmolality
    d. Hyperglycemia, hyperkalemia, alkalosis, elevated serum osmolality

19) You are transporting a 48-year-old male who is complaining of severe epigastric pain that is going through his back. He has been vomiting for the past 8 hours and says that the pain is not improving any. The family says the patient drinks whiskey "constantly". You notice that his skin appears dry and his lips are cracked. Upon palpation of his abdomen, he is very tender and it is distended. He says he cannot get comfortable and keeps turning over. Vitals are as follows: BP 92/54, HR 128, RR 24. What is the next best action for this patient?

    a. Administer antibiotics
    b. Gastric decompression
    c. Administration of fluid and electrolytes
    d. Get patient to the OR

20) Your patient had a recent craniotomy to remove a tumor. He is currently awake, alert and answering your questions appropriately. He shows no signs of any neurologic deficits. His vitals are currently: BP 112/76, HR 88, RR 18/min, O2 @ 97% on 2L, FSBG 96 mg/dL. Since the craniotomy, he has been urinating approximately 50 mL/hr. Within the last couple of hours, his urine output has increased to 350 mL/hr and has a specific gravity of 1.001. What would you suspect?

    a. Development of type 2 diabetes mellitus
    b. Diabetes insipidus
    c. SIADH
    d. Hypervolemia

21) A 54-year-old male has developed diabetes insipidus (DI) after undergoing a craniotomy for a tumor. What findings would you anticipate with this patient?

    a. Oliguria, high serum osmolality, hypernatremia, and low urine specific gravity
    b. Oliguria, low serum osmolality, hyponatremia, and high urine specific gravity
    c. Polyuria, high serum osmolality, hypernatremia, and low urine specific gravity
    d. Polyuria, low serum osmolality, hyponatremia, and high urine specific gravity

22) You are called to transfer a 31-year-old male who sustained extensive electrical burns. Upon entering the room, you notice brown urine in his foley bag. Upon examining the urinalysis, you note myoglobinuria. To prevent the development of acute tubular necrosis and further renal failure, what do you anticipate doing for this patient?

    a. LR, administer hydrochlorothiazide and dobutamine
    b. NS, administer bicarbonate and mannitol
    c. Colloids, administer Lasix and dopamine
    d. NS, administer Lasix and mannitol

23) When treating a septic patient, the flight team knows that the target CVP for fluid resuscitation for a patient with chronic HTN is?

    a. 3-6
    b. 6-10
    c. 8-12
    d. 12-15

24) The flight team knows that when treating a patient with severe sepsis, monitoring the CVP, MAP, urine output, and SvO2 are essential for identifying endpoints for resuscitation. What is the goal for the Sv02 in these severe sepsis patients?

    a. 40-50
    b. 55-65
    c. 65-70
    d. 75-80

25) The flight crew responds to a local small facility for a 21-year-old female being transferred to a level 1 ICU. The patient was involved in an ATV accident with a diagnosis of acute tubular necrosis (ATN) secondary to the crush injuries she experienced when the ATV pinned her against the tree. What would be the most common explanation for the ATN development?

    a. Hypovolemia
    b. Hemorrhage
    c. Hyperkalemia
    d. Rhabomyolysis

26) Which of the following best describes multiple organ dysfunction syndrome (MODS)?

    a. Loss of function of two or more components of the same organ system
    b. Progressive insufficiency of two or more organ systems
    c. Severe septic shock with a lactate greater that 10
    d. Cessation of function of two or more organ systems

27) The flight crew responds to a rural ER for a 29-year-old male that was brought in by local EMS for esophageal varices and upper GI bleed. The patient has an estimated blood loss of 1200 mL. On arrival, the patient informs you he has been drinking since he was 16 years old. The referring RN states that they have established a vasopressin drip and the patient is now complaining of severe chest pain. What would be your first differential diagnosis?

    a. Pneumomediastinum
    b. Mesenteric ischemia
    c. Acute coronary syndrome
    d. Mallory Weiss tear

FlightBridgeED, LLC

28) You respond to a rural med-surg unit to transfer a 61 year-old female with a diagnosis of pneumonia. The referring provider made the decision to transfer the patient due to deterioration throughout the night. The referring RN states that the patient is febrile, tachycardic, tachypneic and has increasing confusion and decreased LOC. The flight crew knows that the initial response of the cardiovascular system to sepsis is:

    a. Increased CVP
    b. Decreased contractility
    c. Increased CI
    d. Bradycardia

29) You have a 13 year-old male patient with a history of insulin dependent diabetes. She is admitted to the local ICU. Her friends and family state that she has had a cold over the past week and has become lethargic over the last 24 hours. Lab results are as follows: Na+ 150, Cl- 103, Glucose 504, WBC 12.3, Band 14%, Leukocytes 68%. The most likely cause of this patient's DKA is:

    a. Acute infection
    b. Dehydration
    c. Noncompliance with insulin
    d. Pancreatitis

30) You are transporting a 50 YOM from the ICU to another facility for further evaluation. The patient has been diagnosed with an AMI. He has been complaining of increasing chest pain, SOB and weight loss. He appears very nervous and you note tremors. His ECG shows atrial fib @ 148. This patient may be experiencing:

    a. Addison's disease
    b. Thyrotoxicosis
    c. Myxedema coma
    d. Cushing's Syndrome

31) You are transporting a patient with a diagnosis of DKA. Current labs and ABGs are as follows: Na+ 140, Cl- 95, Albumin 3.5, K+ 2.4. ABG's: pH 6.9, PCO2 20, HCO3 15, PO2 80, Base deficit -8. Pt has not received any fluid replacement. What is the relationship between pH and K+?

    a. An increase in pH of 0.15 causes an increase in K+ of 0.6
    b. An increase in pH of 0.10 causes a decrease in K+ of 0.6
    c. An increase in pH of 0.08 causes a increase in K+ by 0.20
    d. An increase in pH of 0.10 causes a increase in K+ by 0.08

32) Which of the following ABG's would you suspect to see in a patient that is diagnosed with DKA?

    a. pH 7.40, PaO2 80, PaCO2 30, HCO3 22
    b. pH 7.40, PaO2 70, PaCO2 22, HCO3 33
    c. pH 7.27, PaO2 90, PaCO2 50, HCO3 20
    d. pH 7.20, PaO2 88, PaCO2 23, HCO3 16

33) Black and blue bleeding around the umbilicus is called?

    a. Kehr's sign
    b. Cullen's sign
    c. McBurney's point
    d. Grey-Turners sign

34) The drug of choice for treating a GI bleed is:

    a. Normal saline
    b. Nipride
    c. Sandostatin
    d. Pepcid

35) When treating a patient with suspected DKA, what values would you use to differentiate the diagnosis of DKA from hyperosmolar hyperglycemic nonketotic (HHNK) condition?

    a. A serum glucose of 550 mg/dL
    b. A serum potassium of 3.5 mEq/L
    c. Positive serum ketones
    d. A serum osmolality of 320 mOsm/L

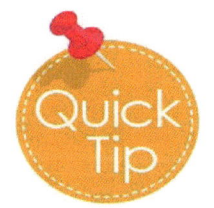

The key-identifying marker used to diagnose DKA vs HHNK is the presence of ketones. The gluconeogenesis causes the incomplete breakdown of free fatty acids, which result in ketones in the blood and urine. HHNK does not have full insulin depletion. No gluconeogenesis takes place. As such no ketones are formed. HHNK will also often have a higher blood glucose level than DKA.

Chapter 12 | Trauma Management

1) Beck's Triad has all of the following EXCEPT?

    a. JVD
    b. Muffled heart tones
    c. Left shoulder pain
    d. Narrowing pulse pressures

2) Newton's 3rd law states?

    a. For every action there is an equal and opposite reaction
    b. An object in motion stays in motion; an object at rest stays at rest
    c. F = MA
    d. None of the above

3) You are transporting a patient that has been involved in a T-Bone type accident. The patient was a restrained driver that was struck on the driver's side. The patient had a brief LOC and is now conversing with you with a GCS of 15. The patient is c/o of left shoulder pain. This is described as?

    a. Chvostek's sign
    b. Kehr's sign
    c. McBurney's Point
    d. Cullen's sign

4) The consensus formula calculates hourly fluid replacement for burn patients. What equation would you use?

    a. 2mL x kg x % BSA
    b. 4mL x kg x % BSA
    c. 6mL x kg x % BSA
    d. 1-3mL x kg x % BSA

5) Minimum urine output for the adult burn patient with non-suspected rhabdomyolysis would be?

    a. 1-5mL/hr
    b. 10-20mL/hr
    c. 30-50mL/hr
    d. 60-80mL/hr

6) You have a 70 KG female patient involved in an MVC that caught fire. She has received first-degree burns to her abdomen and lower back and second and third degree burns to her face, head, hands and both arms. What would you calculate her BSA burns as?

a. 27%
b. 32%
c. 39%
d. 63%

7) You are caring for a male burn patient weighing 120kg with 45% BSA of second and third degree burns. Using the modified formula, what would your fluid resuscitation amount be for the first 8 hours?

a. 6,300-12,600 mL
b. 12,500-25,000 mL
c. 5,400-10,800 mL
d. 4,800-9,600 mL

8) Which of the following is not a treatment strategy when dealing with rhabdomyolosis and myoglobinuria?

a. Mannitol
b. NaHCO3- treatment
c. Fluid resuscitation
d. Vasopressin administration

9) You are managing a burn patient who weighs 90kg with 65% BSA of 2nd and 3rd degree burns. How much fluid should this patient receive in the first 8 hours when using the Parkland formula?

a. 23,400 mL
b. 11,700 mL
c. 8,500 mL
d. 5,850 mL

FlightBridgeED, LLC

10) You are called on a rotor flight to Ohio to pick up a 70kg burn patient that has 45% 2nd and 3rd degree burns. The patient was burned approximately 26 hours ago. The physician reports that the patient has had a total of six liters of fluid in a 24-hour period because he does not want the patient to get cerebral edema. Using the Parkland Formula, how much fluid should this patient have received in the first 24 hours of burn care?

    a. 6,300 mL
    b. 9,450 mL
    c. 12.600 mL
    d. 12,000 mL

11) During transport of a burn patient, you notice an absent P wave and an increased QRS interval on the ECG. Initial ECG showed ST in the 160's with peaked T wave. What electrolyte abnormality do you suspect?

    a. Hypomagnesemia
    b. Hyperkalemia
    c. Hypercalcemia
    d. Hypokalemia

12) Your are transporting a 72 kg male presenting with 2nd and 3rd degree burns to his entire face, anterior torso and complete left arm. How much fluid should the patient get in the first 8 hours using the Parkland formula?

    a. 4,536 mL
    b. 9,200 mL
    c. 2,300 mL
    d. 3,066 mL

13) You are toned for a scene flight for an MVC involving a semi truck versus a car. On arrival, you find an 18 year-old male patient in the front seat with agonal respirations. Prior to extrication, the patient becomes pulseless and apneic. The most common cause of mortality with this type of accident is an aortic tear. An aortic tear is commonly associated with which of the following?

    a. Blunt force injury to the chest wall
    b. Penetration injury to the chest wall
    c. Acceleration/deceleration injury
    d. Cardiac contusion

14) Sudden cardiac death associated with high-speed projectile objects are described as commotio cordis. This is a result of which of the following?

    a. Cardiac tamponade
    b. Cardiac contusion
    c. Fatal dysrhythmia
    d. Aortic arch tear

15) A 24 year-old male presents to his local ER via EMS after an MVC. He is cool, clammy and pale with obvious abdominal distention and pain with palpation, which he rates as 10/10. His current BP is 78/52 and HR 140. He complains of LUQ pain and associated left shoulder pain. He also complains of increased pain with inspiration. The flight nurse notes Cullen's sign upon inspection. What is the most likely cause of his shoulder pain?

    a. Cholelithiasis
    b. Aortic arch tear
    c. Ruptured spleen
    d. Pulmonary contusion

16) Recommended urinary output when caring for an adult patient trauma or medical patient should be?

    a. 100 mL/hr
    b. 30-50 mL/hr
    c. 1-2 mL/hr
    d. > 250mL/hr

17) You are transporting a patient with a history of seizure activity just PTA. The patient has been outside fishing in mid-July. Her husband drove her to the closest ER for treatment. Labs reveal: CK 28,000, BUN 68, CR 2.0, Coags normal and urine is very dark with an output of 20 ml over that past 2 hours. She is unresponsive with a BP 100/40, HR 140, RR 28, and SaO2 of 94%. Your diagnosis is:

    a. TCA overdose
    b. Cushings syndrome
    c. Thyroid storm
    d. Rhabdomyolysis

18) When treating rhabdomyolysis, the flight crewmember knows that giving large amounts of fluid and administering _____ will help by alkalinizing the urine.

    a. Lasix
    b. K+
    c. NaCl-
    d. NaHCO3-

19) The hallmark indicator that rhabdomyolosis is occurring in a hyperthermic patient is?

    a. Altered mental status
    b. Increased BUN
    c. Hyperthermia
    d. Elevated (CK)

20) A 27-year-old multiple trauma patient from the emergency department undergoes fluid resuscitation with 3 L of normal saline solution and 5 units of unwarmed packed red blood cells. He remains unconscious, intubated, and ventilated with 100% oxygen. He has received sedation and remains immobilized on a backboard. The flight nurse should remain concerned about:

    a. Decreased clotting times due to the banked PRBC's
    b. Alkalosis due to the blood administration
    c. Hypothermia due to unwarmed blood
    d. Hypokalemia due to blood administration

21) You are on the scene of a 21 YOM gunshot wound to the left chest. The left chest has been decompressed with a needle. The patient is intubated and continues to de-saturate and you note an increase in SQ air. How will you manage this patient?

    a. Re-needle the left chest
    b. Advance the ETT below the level of the injury
    c. Insert a chest tube
    d. Decrease respiratory rate down to 10 per minute

22) Myoglobinuria, if left untreated, will result in what critical condition?

    a. Hyperkalemic crisis
    b. Acute tubular necrosis
    c. Cardiomyopathy
    d. Polycystic kidney disease

23) When administering PRBC's, the Flight Paramedic can expect a rise in hemoglobin and hematocrit of _____ for each unit of blood?

    a. 1gm/dL increase in the hemoglobin and 3% increase in the hematocrit
    b. 2gm/dL increase in the hemoglobin and a 3% increase in the hematocrit
    c. 1gm/dL increase in the hemoglobin and a 5% increase in the hematocrit
    d. 2gm/dL increase in the hemoglobin and a 5% increase in the hematocrit

24) You are dispatched to an intra-facility transfer to a Level 1 trauma center for a 16 year-old-female with massive head, chest and abdominal trauma from an MVC. She has received 5 units of PRBCs prior to your arrival. She continues to bleed profusely from all of her wounds despite direct pressure to control bleeding and a hypovolemic state. You suspect DIC. What treatment do you expect to administer?

    a. Dobutamine
    b. PRBCs
    c. Rapid fluid volume replacement
    d. Platelets, cryoprecipitate, and FFP

25) You respond to a rural facility to transport a 12 YOM patient with head, chest and thoracic spine trauma. Upon viewing the X-ray, you note a widened mediastinum, obliteration of the aortic knob and the presence of a pleural cap. You suspect what injury?

    a. Tension pneumothorax
    b. Esophageal disruption
    c. Aortic disruption
    d. Tracheal bronchial disruption

26) A massive hemothorax in an adult is defined as a rapid accumulation of more than?

    a. 500cc of blood
    b. 1500cc of blood
    c. 2000cc of blood
    d. 750cc of blood

27) When transferring a patient with multiple or massive transfusion, the flight nurse knows administering multiple units of blood may result in citrate toxicity. What electrolyte is indicated to counteract citrate toxicity?

   a. Sodium
   b. Potassium
   c. Magnesium
   d. Calcium

28) Fractures of the 1st-3rd ribs should indicate a high index of suspicion for which injury?

   a. Esophageal rupture
   b. Aortic Dissection
   c. Pulmonary Contusion
   d. Liver laceration

29) When inserting a chest tube, the correct insertion site recommended is?

   a. 3rd ICS mid-clavicular
   b. 4-5th ICS mid-axillary
   c. 5th ICS mid-axillary
   d. 4th ICS anterior axillary

30) You arrive on the scene to manage a fall victim. She presents with a BP of 70/P, HR 60, RR 28, SaO2 96%. EMS reports the patient has a brief LOC, but now has a GCS 14. You note a deformity to the right femur and she is complaining of neck pain. Your diagnosis of this patient is?

   a. Epidural bleed
   b. Hypovolemic shock
   c. Neurogenic shock
   d. Subdural bleed

31) A patient presenting with Beck's triad is most likely experiencing:

   a. Liver laceration
   b. Tension pneumothorax
   c. Increased ICP
   d. Cardiac tamponade

32) Long-term complications associated with musculoskeletal injuries include all of the following EXCEPT:

   a. Infection
   b. Thrombophlebitis
   c. Delayed bone healing
   d. ARDS

33) Injury patterns associated with rear impact collisions are?

   a. T12/L1 and C-spine fractures
   b. Clavicle, ribs, femur, tib/fib injuries and abdominal injuries
   c. C-spine fractures, clavicle and pelvic fractures
   d. Fractured ribs, skull fractures, patella, femur, acetabular fractures and dislocated hip

34) After a multisystem trauma occurs, death within minutes is usually a result of?

   a. Multisystem organ failure
   b. Blood loss secondary to pelvic fracture
   c. Great vessel laceration
   d. Head injury

35) A 23-year-old male sustained numerous injuries after falling from a roof. You receive report from the transferring RN and are told that the patient has a right tension pneumothorax. Upon assessment, you expect to find?

   a. Tracheal deviation toward the right and diminished or absent breath sounds on the right
   b. Tracheal deviation toward the right and diminished or absent breath sounds on the left
   c. Tracheal deviation toward the left and diminished or absent breath sounds on the left
   d. Tracheal deviation toward the left and diminished or absent breath sounds on the right

36) Of the following, what is the most common cause of myocardial contusion?

   a. Hit to the chest from a high-speed projectile
   b. Getting kicked in the chest by a horse
   c. Injuries after a motor vehicle collision
   d. Performing CPR

37) A 21-year-old female was involved in a domestic disturbance and has several fractured ribs on the (L) side and multiple abrasions and bruising noted on the back and abdomen. She has started to complain of sharp pain in her (L) shoulder. What do you suspect?

    a. Rotator cuff injury
    b. Ruptured spleen
    c. Pulmonary contusion
    d. Thoracic spine injury

38) You are transporting a 32-year-old female who was involved in an MVC with chest trauma. You note Beck's triad and suspect cardiac tamponade. What is included in Beck's triad?

    a. Tachycardia, flat neck veins, muffled heart sounds
    b. Hypertension, distended neck veins, pulsus paradoxus
    c. Hypotension, distended neck veins, muffled heart sounds
    d. Hypotension, flat neck veins, decreased right atrial pressure

39) You are called to transfer a 23 YO male patient that was involved in a head-on accident with a semi-truck. The patient is currently showing s/s of hypoxia with a NRB @ 15 L/min being administered. Currently the patient has a GCS of 10 and breathing shallow and rapid @ 28 / min. Current labs and V/S: BP 100/70, P 139, RR 28, Skin pale/dry/warm. H & H - 7 & 19. The patient has a current urine output of 0.5mL/kg/hr for the past 3 hours. What type of shock is the patient suffering from?

    a. Hypoxic hypoxia
    b. Stagnant hypoxia
    c. Hypemic hypoxia
    d. Histotoxic hypoxia

40) You respond to an inter-facility transfer for a 21 YO female that is being transferred for respiratory distress. The patient sustained a pulmonary contusion in a MVC. She has no medical history or pulmonary disease. Over the past few hours she has been complaining of worsening dyspnea, with her respiratory rate increasing and her SaO2 decreasing. Breath sounds reveal fine crackles bilaterally. Her ABGs reveal a respiratory alkalosis with an associated hypoxemia. The chest x-ray shows patchy infiltrates. She is diagnosed with ARDS. Because of her hypoxia, high flow oxygen is applied and ABGs are trended. Considering the high concentration of oxygen this patient is requiring to maintain an adequate SaO2, close assessment for clinical indication of oxygen toxicity is important. Which of the following will manifest first with this condition?

        a. Moist, productive cough
        b. Substernal chest pain
        c. Dyspnea
        d. Cyanosis

41) You are called to transfer a 21 YO patient from a small regional facility to a level 1 trauma center. Prior to your arrival, the referring MD has placed a pulmonary artery catheter to monitor the patient's hemodynamic status. During report you note that the patient has had significant changes in the past 6 hours. He is febrile with a temp of 101.4 F, skin is warm and dry and the patient seems restless and agitated. His current hemodynamic parameters are: BP 84/38, HR 134, CO 10.1, CI 5.2, CVP 4.2, PCWP 4, SVR 452, SvO2 90%. What does the high SvO2 reading indicate?

        a. Intra-cardiac shunt
        b. Increased oxygen delivery
        c. Severe hypoxia
        d. Decreased oxygen extraction

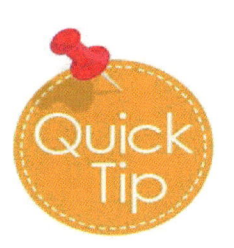

Quick Tip

Permissive hypotension is the standard of care now in trauma management. Massive fluid resuscitation has been shown to start the DIC and inflammatory process. In addition, raising the MAP above 65 mmHg will cause an increase in bleeding to the blunt or penetrating trauma patients.

FlightBridgeED, LLC

Chapter 13 | Neurological Emergencies

1) Your patient has the following hemodynamic parameters: BP 170/80, HR 60, RR 22 & irregular, ICP 23, CVP 20, PA 32/14, PCWP 15. What's your patients CPP?

    a. 46
    b. 52
    c. 87
    d. 81

2) Brown–Sequard Syndrome is a rare spinal cord injury that involves?

    a. Anterior cord lesions
    b. Posterior cord lesions
    c. Central cord lesions
    d. Ipsilateral cord lesions

3) You're dispatched to a scene flight at night for a possible man that has fallen off a bridge. On arrival you find that your patient was involved from a fall of 20'. EMS states that he had a brief loss of consciousness and a period of lucidness, but now is fading in and out of consciousness. This presentation most often presents with what type of head trauma?

    a. Epidural bleed
    b. Intraventricular bleed
    c. Subdural bleed
    d. Diffuse axonal injury

4) Cushing's Triad consists of?

    a. Widening pulse pressures, tachycardia and normal respirations
    b. Hypertension, bradycardia and respiratory changes (Cheyne Stokes)
    c. Hypotension, widening pulse pressures, bradycardia
    d. Hypertension, tachycardia, narrowing pulse pressures

5) Diffuse axonal injury will most likely represent how on a CT scan?

   a. Normal and unidentifiable
   b. Granulated or salt and pepper appearance
   c. Identified by cervical spine subluxation
   d. All the above

6) Your patient has an ICP of 28. The current BP is 100/60. HIs cerebral perfusion pressure is approximately?

   a. 45 mmHg
   b. 60 mmHg
   c. 70-90 mmHg
   d. 100 mmHg

7) A 60 year-old female patient with a history of extensive emphysema became unresponsive while watching TV with her husband. Local EMS transported the patient to the local ED where you are called to transport the patient to a level 1-stroke center. On your primary assessment, you note paralysis of her left extremities, aphasia, and decreased LOC with a current GCS of 12. Which of the following would be a contraindication to fibrinolytics?

   a. Seizure
   b. Sluggish, dilated pupils
   c. Cholecystectomy 6 months ago
   d. Abdominal aortic aneurysm

8) Normal adult CPP is at least?

   a. 40 mmHg
   b. 60 mmHg
   c. 70 mmHg
   d. 50 mmHg

9) You respond to a rural facility to pick up a patient with a diagnosis of a skull fracture. Upon arrival, the x-ray shows multiple fractures that radiate from a compressed area. What type of skull fracture does this patient have?

   a. Basilar fracture
   b. Linear stellate fracture
   c. Diastatic fracture
   d. Depressed skull fracture

10) Calculate the following cerebral perfusion pressure?

BP 150/75, HR 140, RR 28, SaO2 100%, CVP 2, ICP 25

  a. 98
  b. 65
  c. 75
  d. 125

11) When evaluating the CT of a patient believed to have a diffuse axonal injury you expect to see?

  a. A contact lens shaped collection of blood
  b. An unremarkable CT scan
  c. A large collection of blood covering a single hemisphere
  d. High density region surrounded by zones of low density

12) The classic description of a patient suffering from an epidural hematoma is?

  a. Rapid onset of unconsciousness, posturing and seizure
  b. Unconsciousness, followed by a brief period of lucidity, and a period of rapid decrease in the level of consciousness
  c. Slow loss of consciousness, pupillary changes, and seizures
  d. Slow loss of consciousness, ipsilateral posturing, and contralateral pupillary changes

13) A basilar skull fracture is associated with all of the following EXCEPT:

  a. CSF rhinorrhea
  b. CSF otorrhea
  c. Seventh cranial nerve palsy
  d. Eleventh cranial nerve paralysis

14) When monitoring invasive intracranial pressure lines, the transducer should be leveled at the?

  a. Foramen of Kellie
  b. Foramen of Ovale
  c. Foramen of Monro
  d. Foramen of Magnum

15) The patient suffering from Brown-Sequard Syndrome presents with which of the following S/S?

    a. Complete flaccidity below the level of the injury
    b. Ipsilateral motor loss, contralateral pain loss
    c. Greater weakness in upper extremities than in lower extremities
    d. Complete motor pain and temperature loss below the level of the injury

16) You are flying a 56 YO female secondary to a severe headache that came on suddenly. She states that she's been out of her blood pressure medication for 3 weeks and cannot afford to buy more. Her blood pressure ranges from 250/138 to 210/126. The referring MD has started Nitroprusside and oxygen by NRB. Which of the following describes appropriate drug therapy and goals for this patient presentation.

    a. Beta blockers to decrease contractility
    b. Arterial vasodilators to decrease afterload
    c. Diuretics to decrease preload
    d. Venous vasodilators to decrease preload

17) The flight team is dispatched for a transfer at the local ER for a patient that's suffering from a Sub-Arachnoid Hemorrhage. What is the goal for systolic blood pressure for this patient during transport?

    a. 120 systolic
    b. 130 systolic
    c. 140 systolic
    d. 160 systolic

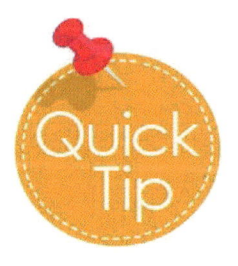

It's essential to maintain a MAP pressure between 85-90 mmHg so as to perfuse the brain as well as the kidneys. CPP needs to be at least 70 mmHg. To identify a CPP, the formula is: MAP - ICP. You're not going to know the patients current ICP so use the upper end of the normal range. Normal range is 0-15 mmHg.

FlightBridgeED, LLC
Chapter 14 | Toxicology

1) You are transporting a patient who consumed a significant overdose of Elavil (amitriptyline). Upon your assessment, you would expect to find what patient presentation?

    a. Bradycardia and hypotension
    b. Hyperventilation and hyporeflexia
    c. Fever and agitation
    d. Severe bradycardia and salivation

2) You arrive on scene to find a 53-year old female who overdosed on nevibolol (Bystolic) as a suicide attempt. On the monitor, you notice this:

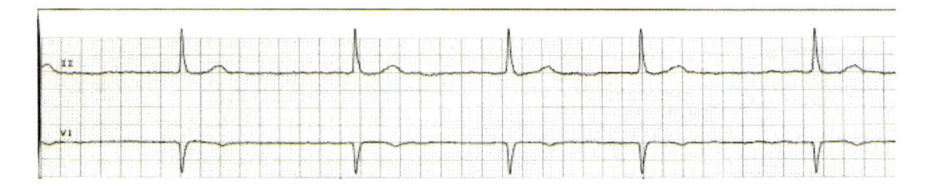

Which of the following therapies would be anticipated to be unsuccessful?

    a. Dopamine
    b. Transcutaneous Pacing
    c. Atropine
    d. Glucagon IVP

3) You are transporting a patient who ingested an unknown substance. On assessment, the patient is unconscious and you obtain the following EKG:

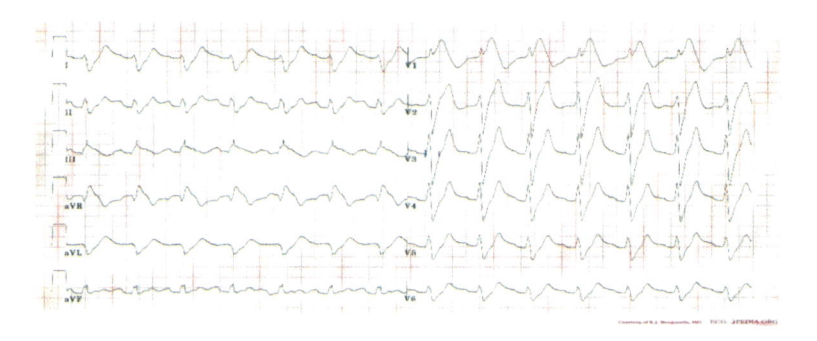

You suspect an OD related to what substance:

    a. Paxil (paroxetine)
    b. Pamelor (nortriptyline)
    c. Tenormin (atenolol)
    d. Digoxin (digitalis)

4) You arrive at a facility to transport a patient who says they took an entire bottle of acetaminophen (Tylenol). They are currently complaining of RUQ pain. Based on this presentation, when did this patient most likely ingest this drug:

    a. Less than one hour ago
    b. Within the last 1-4 hours
    c. Within the last 6-12 hours
    d. Within the last 24-72 hours

5) You are treating an 86 year old male with digitalis toxicity due to an accidental overdose. What electrolyte would be evaluated first with this known diagnosis?

    a. Calcium
    b. Potassium
    c. Sodium
    d. Chloride

6) You have a patient who received an unintentional overdose of potassium after a medication error occurred. His current K+ is 7.84, pH is 7.35 and his current ECG is:

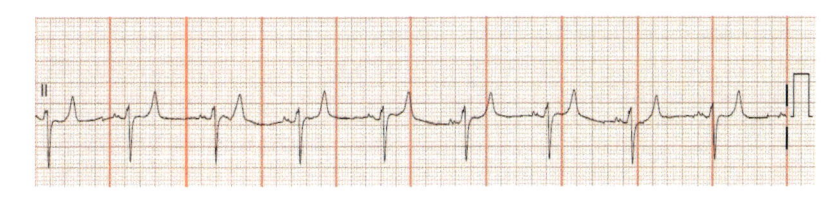

How would you manage this patient? What medications would you anticipate providing?

1.
2.
3.
4.
5.

7) Your patient was exposed to cyanide. What antidote management would best suit this patient?

   a. Physostigmine
   b. Oxygen
   c. Atropine and 2-PAM
   d. Amyl nitrate and sodium thiosulfate

8) In an aspirin overdose, the primary acid base disturbance would be _____ followed by _____ ?

   a. Respiratory alkalosis; metabolic acidosis
   b. Respiratory acidosis; metabolic acidosis
   c. Respiratory alkalosis; metabolic alkalosis
   d. Respiratory acidosis; metabolic alkalosis

9) Which medication could potentially prevent the early symptoms of hypoglycemia?

   a. Valium
   b. Verapamil
   c. Metoprolol
   d. Lisinopril

10) A 37 year-old male patient is being transferred to a higher level ICU secondary to an overdose from an unknown drug. During your primary assessment, you note the patient is very thin. Upon obtaining an EKG, you note a prolonged QT segment. Based on your understanding of pathophysiology, you would anticipate a reduction in a certain electrolyte that may be causing these problems. Which electrolyte is least likely to be the cause of the prolonged QT?

   a. Magnesium
   b. Calcium
   c. Potassium
   d. Sodium

11) You are transporting a patient who overdosed on her prescription medication. Within minutes of your transport, you notice torsades de pointes on the cardiac monitor. Based upon this rhythm disturbance, what medication do you suspect the patient ingested?

    a. Fluoxetine (Prozac)
    b. Metoprolol (Lopressor)
    c. Hydrocodone (Lortab)
    d. Amitriptyline (Elavil)

12) Your patient has a diagnosis of salicylate toxicity. What acid-base imbalances would you anticipate?

    a. Respiratory alkalosis and metabolic acidosis
    b. Respiratory alkalosis and metabolic alkalosis
    c. Respiratory acidosis and metabolic acidosis
    d. Respiratory acidosis and metabolic alkalosis

Chapter 15 | OB/GYN Emergencies

1) The term effacement refers to?

    a. Cervical dilation
    b. Position of fetal head
    c. Thickness of cervix and represented as a %
    d. The lie of the baby

2) Your patient is presenting active delivery and you have a breech presentation. Delivery is halted upon delivery of the head. What would be the best next action?

    a. Administer Brethine 0.25mg SQ
    b. Administer MgSO4 4g IV bolus
    c. Perform Mauriceu's Maneuver
    d. Place patient in the knee-chest position

3) Poor variability is caused by all of the following EXCEPT?

    a. Fetal hypoxia
    b. Extreme prematurity
    c. Smoking by mother
    d. Nuchal Cord

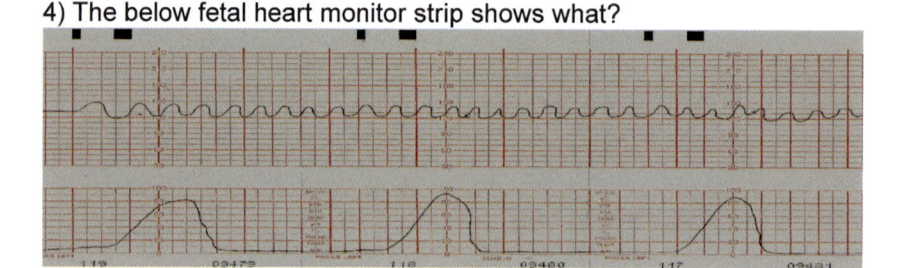

4) The below fetal heart monitor strip shows what?

    a. Sinusoidal
    b. Good variability
    c. Early decels
    d. Accels

5) The most accepted initial treatment for PIH related to hypertension may include all of the following EXCEPT?

   a. Labetalol 10-20mg IVP
   b. Brethine 0.25mg SQ
   c. MgSO4 4-6g slow IVP
   d. Hydralazine 2mg IVP

6) The second stage of labor ends with:

   a. Start of contractions
   b. Delivery of the fetus
   c. Full effacement
   d. Crowning

7) You are transferring a 32-week gestation female to a higher level OB unit. The patient has received a 4 g bolus of MgSO4 and is currently on an infusion drip of 5 g/hr. You assess your patient's DTRs and note they are absent. You discontinue the infusion and recheck DTRs after 5 minutes. You suspect acute MgSO4 toxicity. What would be your treatment?

   a. Brethine 0.25mg SQ
   b. CaCl 1g / 10 mL
   c. Lasix
   d. NaHCO3 50mEq IVP

8) You arrive on the scene of a 21 year-old-female involved in a single rollover accident who is approximately 28 weeks pregnant. The patient is gravida 2, para 1. Your assessment reveals palpation of fetal parts over the abdomen. What is your diagnosis?

   a. Liver laceration
   b. Abruptio placenta
   c. Uterine rupture
   d. Placenta previa

9) The patient is a breech presentation and delivery appears to be halted upon delivery of the head. The appropriate action would be to?

   a. Initiate rapid transport, placing mother in a knee-chest position
   b. Administer tocolytic agents
   c. Perform Trousseau's maneuver
   d. Perform Mauriceau's maneuver

10) Which of the following fetal heart tone tracings is an ominous sign?

   a. Sinusoidal
   b. Early decelerations
   c. Variable decelerations
   d. Accelerations

11) When administering MgSO4 to prevent seizures in the OB patient, therapeutic levels range from 4-8mEq/L. What assessment finding indicates toxic levels for the OB patient?

   a. Elevated BP
   b. Elevated RR
   c. Elevated HR
   d. Absent DTRs

12) HELLP syndrome is characterized by?

   a. Hypertension, elevated liver enzymes and low platelets
   b. Hypertension, elevated lipase and low protein
   c. Hemolysis, elevated liver enzymes and low platelets
   d. Hemolysis, elevated lipase and low protein

13) Postpartum hemorrhage is defined as blood loss of 500cc or greater following delivery. You have attempted vigorous fundal massage without any improvement in bleeding. You should next be considering what?

   a. Administration of PRBCs
   b. Continued vigorous fundal massage
   c. Methergine 0.2mg IM or IV
   d. Pitocin 20-40 units in 1000cc of LR

14) Late decelerations may indicate?

   a. Cord compression
   b. Uterine placental insufficiency
   c. Acidosis
   d. Inadequate uterine contractions

15) What are the three classic s/s of pregnancy induced hypertension (PIH)?

   a. Headache, hyper-reflexia, and HELLP
   b. Hypertension, edema, and proteinuria
   c. Hypertension, headache, and proteinuria
   d. Hypertension, headache, and hyper-reflexia

16) Which of the following maneuvers may be used to help deliver an infant with shoulder dystocia?

   a. Erb's maneuver
   b. Forceps technique maneuver
   c. Leopold's maneuver
   d. McRobert's maneuver

17) A 32 year-old-female who has IDDM and is 30 weeks gestation is going to be transferred to a high risk OB facility. The patient has had contractions every 5 minutes for the last hour and has received one liter of NS. You should prepare to:

   a. Administer 0.25 mg Brethine SQ
   b. Maintain an IV of D5W throughout transport
   c. Verify adequate urine output secondary to your fluid bolus
   d. Administer Magnesium Sulfate 4 g bolus over 20-30 min

18) In evaluating fetal heart characteristics, which is the most important in determining neurological maturity?

   a. Accelerations
   b. Variability
   c. Flat or decreased beat-to-beat variability
   d. Transient accelerations and decelerations from the baseline FHR

19) The flight team recognizes that DIC is a common complication of?

   a. Abruptio placenta
   b. Ovarian rupture
   c. Ectopic pregnancy
   d. Placenta previa

Chapter 16 | Neonatal & Pediatric Emergencies

1) Your patient is reported to have transposition of the great vessels. It is essential to the survival of the neonate to maintain?

   a. Oxygen
   b. PDA patency
   c. Indomethacin
   d. Oxytocin

2) The equation for determination of ETT size in a neonate or child is?

   a. (12+4)/4
   b. 16 X 2)/ 2
   c. (16+age) / 4
   d. (16+age)(4)

3) When giving a neonate PGE1 for PDA patency, the flight crewmember knows that a primary complication to administration is?

   a. Closure of the PDA
   b. Apnea
   c. Pulmonary HTN
   d. Metabolic acidosis

4) With regards to volume loss due to hemorrhage, the flight crewmember knows that the pediatric patient will not demonstrate hypotension until approximately _____ loss of blood volume.

   a. 10%
   b. 30%
   c. 25%
   d. 40%

5) A common injury pattern seen in pediatrics stuck by a vehicle is called?

   a. Beck's triad
   b. Cushing's triad
   c. Waddell's triad
   d. Kehr's sign

6) Your 10kg neonate starts presenting with a repetitive mouth & tongue movement, bicycling motion, eye deviation and rapid blinking. What type of seizure would this represent?

a. Clonic
b. Tonic
c. Myoclonic
d. Subtle

7) A neonate who is experiencing repetitive motion of a bicycling type action with lip smacking is presenting with what type of seizure?

a. Subtle
b. Tonic
c. Clonic
d. Myoclonic

8) The high vascular resistance in the fetal lung is due to the following physiologic mechanisms?

a. Changes in O2 tension
b. Changes in pH and CO2 tension
c. Pulmonary arterial vasoconstriction
d. Increase in systemic vascular resistance

9) During transport of a neonate, which of the following findings would indicate that the neonate is in stress?

a. Sucking
b. Fist clinched
c. Hiccoughing or sneezing
d. Quiet and alert

10) Increased irritability, increased HR and BP, eye fluttering and decreased SaO2 may be subtle signs of?

a. Seizures
b. Congenital heart defect
c. Hydrocephalus
d. Neurological anomaly

FlightBridgeED, LLC

11) You are transporting a 32-week premature neonate with respiratory distress. Which drug may be administered in preparation for transport?

   a. Antibiotics
   b. Surfactant
   c. D10
   d. Prostaglandin

12) Your patient is PDA dependent. This would indicate that your patient would likely require the administration of which of the following drugs?

   a. Indomethacin
   b. Progesterone
   c. Prostaglandin
   d. Synthetic surfactant

13) Which of the following is one of the most common side effects complicating the transport of a neonate receiving prostaglandin therapy?

   a. Hypertension
   b. Hypothermia
   c. Apnea
   d. Tachypnea

14) You are called to transport a 5-day-old neonate. On arrival, your report states that the baby is suffering from tetralogy of fallot. You know that this disease process causes severe hypoxia. What is the long-term treatment to correct the heart defect?

   a. PGE-1 administration
   b. High flow oxygen
   c. Cath and dilate the PA and patch the VSD
   d. Indomethacin for PDA closure

15) Which of the following congenital disorders results in a right to left shunt?

   a. PDA
   b. Isolated VSD
   c. Tetralogy of fallot
   d. ASD

16) The primary stimulus, which causes closure of the PDA, is?

    a. Prostaglandin
    b. Oxygen
    c. Indomethacin
    d. Lasix

17) You are transporting a patient suffering from choanal atresia. You know that your patient will have difficulty with all of the following EXCEPT?

    a. Sleeping
    b. Breathing
    c. Feeding
    d. Diuresis

18) The most common congenital heart defect in neonates is?

    a. Patent ductus arteriosus (PDA)
    b. Aortic stenosis
    c. Tetralogy of fallot
    d. Ventricular septal defect (VSD)

19) When determining ETT size for a 4 year-old-male patient. The flight paramedic calculates the appropriate un-cuffed ETT size to be?

    a. 4.5 ETT
    b. 4.0 ETT
    c. 5.0 ETT
    d. 5.5 ETT

20) When calculating ETT depth of insertion on a 4 YO that has been intubated with a 5.0 ETT, the Flight Nurse knows that an appropriate depth of insertion is?

    a. 10 cm
    b. 11 cm
    c. 15 cm
    d. 18 cm

21) Steeple sign on the AP neck X-ray indicates what pediatric respiratory problem?

   a. Epiglottitis
   b. Croup
   c. Bronchiolitis
   d. Airway obstruction

22) Immediately following RSI and of an 8 yo male, and the use of succinylcholine, this patient develops a widened QRS and then a sinusoidal rhythm on the monitor and goes into cardiopulmonary arrest. What condition do you suspect?

   a. Hypovolemic shock
   b. Anaphylactic shock
   c. Hypoxemia
   d. Hyperkalemic crisis

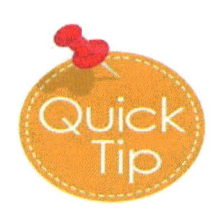

Understanding the different neonatal heart defects and their underlying physiology can be overwhelming. They all share a common trend and have ductal lesions along with other manifestations. However, maintaining a patent ductus is essential. It's the only way your neonate will remain oxygenated. Oxygen is the main way our body responds to close the ductus. Due to this, maintaining the lowest possible FiO2 is important. It's not abnormal to have SaO2 readings in the 70% range throughout the care of the neonate. Prostaglandin is also administered to maintain patency. Apnea is the major side affect and as such, all neonates being given Prostaglandin will need to be intubated and placed on the transport ventilator.

Chapter 17 | Review Question Rationale

Chapter 1 | Oxygenation Pathophysiology

1) **Correct answer: C** This would be partially compensated due to the fact of the PaCO2 being lower than normal with metabolic involvement. The patient is attempting to blow off the acid.
2) **Correct answer: A** This is classic uncompensated respiratory alkalosis because of the pH being high (Alk) and the PaCO2 being low (not enough acid). There is no metabolic compensation. Classic first stage of shock!
3) **Correct answer: D** For every 0.10 increase in pH, you will have a corresponding decrease in K+ by 0.6. Any patient with a critically low K+ should receive runs of 20-40mEq of K+ prior to trying to correct a metabolic disorder (increasing pH).
4) **Correct answer: C** For every change in PCO2 of 10mmHg, you will have a change in pH of 0.08 in the opposite direction. The is an excellent way to correct pH in a patient with an abnormal pH.
5) **Correct answer: A** Remember that with Bohr effect and the presence of increased acid or lower pH, your Hgb will release its load of O2 to the tissues. In a right shift on the oxyhemoglobin curve we see "R" for raised acid, temp, 2-3 DPG and PaO2.
6) **Correct answer: D** Lactate levels will increase in dehydration and muscle excursion. However, it is also the most sensitive marker for tissue perfusion and predicting mortality in sepsis and septic shock. Every point > 2.5 increases mortality by 10%.

7) **Correct answer: C** This is a common question where you will just need to remember the formula. Always remember that any effect in EtCO2 will have an effect in pH in the opposite direction. Formula = 10mmHg change in PaCO2 will have an opposite change in pH of 0.08.
8) **Correct answer: B** Because the pH is still in the compensatory range of 7.35-7.45, this would have a "first name" of compensated. Next, think of your last name. Anything that falls below 7.40 is an acid. So you have the first name of compensated and a last name of Acidosis. Now find the middle name. Next look at the PaCO2. You have a high value meaning you have too much acid. This is the respiratory component. Your HCO3- is in the normal range. There is no kidney involvement. Your middle name is respiratory. This is a compensated respiratory acidosis.
9) **Correct answer: C** Always remember that basic response we have in a stress situation. Our respiratory rate will increase and then our heart rate. This initial RR increase will cause an initial respiratory alkalosis.
10) **Correct answer: B** This again is a recall question. Remember that an increase or decrease of HCO3 of 10mEq will change the pH by 0.15 in the same direction. This response is going to have the biggest impact, as it translates to correcting an abnormal pH.
11) **Correct answer: D** Go through your steps in the ABG diagnosis. Identify the first name. This would be uncompensated because we have a pH that is outside the compensatory range of 7.35-7.45. Current pH is 7.6. Next identify the last name. This would be an Alkalosis because it is > 7.45. Next identify the middle name. Look at the PaCO2. Is it

normal? No! It's lower than the compensatory range of 35-45. So you know that a lower PaCO2 tells you that you're losing acid. Double-check the HCO3. Is it normal? No! Your kidneys are not able to excrete the HCO3-. Your middle name is then mixed. Your correct answer is a mixed disturbance.

12) **Correct answer: B** Remember your rule. A 10mmHg change in PaCO2 will change the pH by 0.08 in the opposite direction. You have a drop of 20mmHg in the EtCO2. This translates to 0.16 in pH increase. Add this to the initial pH and you have a final answer of 7.26.

13) **Correct answer: C** Remember the rules for respiratory failure. You have both of the criteria present. PaCO2 > 50 and associated hypoxia with the PaO2 < 60. This patient is going downhill and needs airway intervention and good ventilator management strategies.

14) **Correct answer: C** Whenever a patient is suffering from metabolic acidosis, there will be a shift of K+ out of the cell and into the blood. Remember that often, this is a false high and should never be treated. Center your treatment around fixing the metabolic acidosis and trend the K+ often to identify changes. The one presentation that would make you focus on treatment of the K+ would be in a DKA patient. DKA patients will either result in a critically low K+ or a normal to high K+. Always give runs of K+ in these patients because of the fluid resuscitation and the correction of the metabolic disorder. You will washout any free K+, so make sure you give K+ and trend labs for desired effect.

15) **Correct answer: D** Because of how the PRBCs are stored and how lack the properties associated with whole blood, rapid massive transfusion will result in depletion of 2-3 DPG and thus move the oxyhemaglobin curve to the left. Remember, a curve to the left causes an increased "affinity", causing Hgb to hold onto O2. This will cause an excellent SaO2 saturation, but a poor PaO2 (tissue hypoxia).
16) **Correct answer: D** Continued O2 suctioning will cause a severe metabolic alkalosis. Metabolic alkalosis is a primary increase in serum bicarbonate (HCO3-) concentration. This occurs as a consequence of a loss of H+ from the body or a gain in HCO3-. In its purest form, it manifests as an alkalemia (pH >7.40). As a compensatory mechanism, metabolic alkalosis leads to alveolar hypoventilation with a rise in arterial carbon dioxide tension (PaCO2), which diminishes the change in pH that would otherwise occur.
17) **Correct answer: A** This patient is suffering from a low PaO2 and lower than desired SaO2. All other ventilator settings are appropriate. By increasing the FiO2 and PEEP you increase oxygenation the quickest.
18) **Correct answer: B** SaO2 is reflective of how much O2 is attached to the Hgb.
19) **Correct answer: C** You should have identified the first name as uncompensated, middle name as metabolic and the last name of acidosis. You also need to look at the PaCO2. It's low and showing that the patient is attempting to compensate for the metabolic disorder by blowing CO2 using the respiratory buffering system. So you should have

identified a partially compensated metabolic acidosis.
20) **Correct answer: C** The classic identifying parameters for diagnosis of acute respiratory failure is PaO2 < 60 and a PaCO2 > 50.
21) **Correct answer: D** Think "R". Shifts to the right are caused from things raised. Remember the definition of the Bohr effect. The Bohr effect states that Hgb will unload its O2 when there is raised acid. The Hgb will have decreased affinity. So you will have a low SaO2 and a high PaO2. So anything raised: 2-3 DPG, hyperthermia, CO2, PaO2 and acid, will cause a right shift.
22) **Correct answer: C** When we think about the left shift, allows think "L" for Low or Left. Decreased 2-3 DPG, hypothermia, low CO2 and low PaO2 will cause the Hgb to hold on to O2. This causes a higher affinity. You will see a great SaO2 and a poor PaO2 leading to a false sense of oxygenation. You think the patient is oxygenating fine, when actually the patient has tissue hypoxia.
23) **Correct answer: C** While giving patients massive transfusion secondary to hemorrhage, the flight clinician needs to understand that guiding overall resuscitation on blood replacement is wrong. Resuscitation should be guided on lactate and base deficit levels. While giving many units of PRBCs, the patient can become hypothermic. In addition, the citrate added to the PRBCs kill off the 2-3 DPG. This causes the Hgb to lose the ability to release oxygen to the tissues and drives the oxyhemoglobin curve to the left. This in turn causes cellular hypoxia. We think by giving PRBCs that we are increasing oxygen carrying capacity, but we can cause other issues if not careful. The second aspect

to consider would be to give prophylactic Ca++ replacement as well. Remember, citrate binds with Ca++ and magnesium and causes the patient to have decreased levels. By giving the Ca++, you will increase SVR and help with contractility in the shock patient.

24) **Correct answer: D** When understanding the oxyhemoglobin dissociation curve, the clinician knows that pH, 2,3-DPG levels, body temperature, and massive transfusion with PRBCs all play a significant role in hemoglobin's affinity or lack of for oxygen. Cardiac output plays no direct role in this phenomenon.

25) **Correct answer: B** The bicarbonate buffering system is important in the acid-base homeostasis of the body. In this system, CO2 combines with H2O to form carbonic acid (H2CO3). This rapidly dissociates to form hydrogen ions and bicarbonate (HCO3-).

26) **Correct answer: C** Hydrogen ions will cause a state of acidosis. All other choices will lead to a state of alkalosis.

27) **Correct answer: D** In the early (hyperdynamic) phase of septic shock, oxygen delivery is increased but the tissues cannot extract and use the oxygen, therefore the consumption is decreased and the venous oxygen saturation would be increased. Lactic acidosis will ensue because the cells become hypoxic from not being able to utilize the oxygen.

28) **Correct answer: A** This formula is the standard in the critical care environment to identify how much oxygen is delivered per minute as well as how much oxygen is dissolved in the plasma. Remember that 98% of oxygen is bound to Hgb, with the remainder dissolved in the plasma. The body uses the stored oxygen in the plasma first, and then if needed, pulls oxygen from the hemoglobin. This formula is great to use in conjunction with the Fick formula as well as to trend the SvO2, and compare that with the

amount delivered. In most sepsis patients, supply and demand are not equal, with the demand often exceeding the supply.

29) **Correct answer: A** In this patient scenario, the patient is suffering from acidosis and is febrile. Remember a right shift is "Right" for the patient. All things are "R"aised. temperature, acid, 2-3 DPG and PaO2. Bohr effect states that in the presence of increased acid, the Hgb will have less of an affinity to oxygen. This means that the Hgb molecules dump off the loads of oxygen to the tissues instead of storing oxygen like normal. In an acidotic state, we build an abundance of H+ ions and CO2. Those now take a seat on the Hgb molecule and don't leave any room for oxygen to be stored. This results in good tissue oxygenation, high PO2 and a low SaO2.

30) **Correct answer: D** With any patient that receives massive PRBC transfusions, they will become depleted of platelets. Often, the standard rule is for every 5 units of PRBCs, you would administer 1 unit of platelets. In addition, most level 1 facilities will give FFP instead of platelets.

31) **Correct answer: B** Because of the citrate that is used to preserve the PRBCs, the citrate binds with calcium and magnesium and causes the patient to have hypocalcaemia. The citrate also kills the 2-3 DPG. This is what causes the patient's oxyhemoglobin curve to shift to the left. The 2-3 DPG is the crowbar that pops off the O2 molecule from the Hgb. If this important aspect is depleted, tissue oxygenation will become worse. Any patient that receives massive transfusion protocols, requires optimal oxygenation resuscitation, and is essential because of this phenomenon.

FlightBridgeED, LLC
Chapter 2 | Respiratory Emergencies

1) **Correct answer: C** Decadron is a corticosteroid used to decrease inflammation. Albuterol, terbutaline, and ketamine all have bronchodilating effects when administered.
2) **Correct answer: B** COPD patients will develop polycythemia in response to hypoxia as a means of attempting to compensate. The same concept that increases RBC production also increases 2-3 DPG production.
3) **Correct answer: D** A shift in the trachea away from the needle would indicate a worsening tension pneumothorax with greater tracheal deviation. All other choices are indicators of improvement after the procedure is performed.
4) **Correct answer: C** Tingling and sensory changes are not an anticipated finding or side effect from the administration of Albuterol. All other findings are commonly seen after the medication has been administered.
5) **Correct answer: B** Ground glass opacities can indicate many things including infection, pulmonary edema and cellular inflammation. Look at the presentation. There is no indication of pulmonary edema or CHF. This in early onset and only identified due to the chest film and the decreasing PaO2.
6) **Correct answer: A** PCP is a form of pneumonia, caused by a fungus. It is considered an opportunistic infection, and seen especially in those patients with cancer, HIV/AIDS, or a weak immune system.

7) **Correct answer: D** Ketamine has bronchodilating properties and is useful in asthma patients. Using IV ketamine will result in general anesthesia without significant respiratory depression. Bronchodilation begins within minutes of administering the medication and lasts approximately 20-30 minutes after cessation of the medication. In addition, ketamine has great analgesic effects along with sedative effects and is very good with patients that have hemodynamic instability.
8) **Correct answer: C** In patients with reactive airway disease, such as those with asthma or sometimes COPD, using non-cardio selective beta-blockers may cause bronchospasm. For patients with reactive airway disease, administration blocks the beta-2 receptors and can cause worsening of their condition.
9) **Correct answer: C** Alveolar dead space occurs with no perfusion with ventilation. Intrapulmonary shunt would occur when there is no perfusion or ventilation. A pulmonary embolus will cause the patient to hyperventilate, causing them to become very fatigued.
10) **Correct answer: A** Sepsis is the most common cause of ARDS secondary to the release of inflammatory cytokines and the break down of the alveolar-capillary membrane. Inhalation of harmful substances, such as smoke or chemical fumes, severe pneumonia, and head or chest injury, can also lead to the development of ARDS.
11) **Correct answer: B** Fluctuation in the water-seal chamber indicates that the tube is patent and positioned correctly. When a patient is spontaneously breathing, inspiration is

negative pressure and causes the water levels to rise. Upon expiration, the pressure is positive and causes the water levels to fall. If the patient is being mechanically ventilated, inspiration is positive and the water level would fall, and expiration is neutral and the water level would rise.

12) **Correct answer: C** Respiratory acidosis results from an increase in the PaCO2. The best way to overcome this is to decrease the PaCO2 by improving overall minute ventilation.

13) **Correct answer: B** The most common cause would be atelectasis, which is common after surgery and especially in smokers. This patient needs to deep breath and use incentive spirometry to improve ventilation and prevent pneumonia from occurring.

14) **Correct answer: C** A significant elevation in lactate indicates multi-system involvement and is associated with a poor prognosis in these patients. LDH catalyzes the conversion of pyruvate and lactate with the conversion of NADH in the Krebs cycle when in anaerobic metabolism. It's essentially a feedback loop and sends signals that the lack of oxygen stops ATP production and the glycolysis phase takes over for ATP (2) production. An elevated fever and leukocytosis indicate an infection but not necessarily an indicator of a poorer prognosis.

15) **Correct answer: B** Recall that approximately 97% of oxygen is attached to Hgb, so SaO2 is a more accurate reading of the amount of oxygen in the blood. The PaO2 represents only about 3% of the oxygen dissolved in the plasma. When measuring CO, it is a reflection of how well the heart is pumping the blood with the hemoglobin and oxygen attached. The SvO2 is associated with the oxygen reserve and is what is left over after the tissues have extracted

the oxygen they need. The MAP is a calculation reflecting organ tissue perfusion but does not have any indication regarding the amount of oxygen in the blood.

16) **Correct answer: C** Patients with a diagnosis of pulmonary embolus display tachypnea and dyspnea, which leads to a state of respiratory alkalosis. This would cause an increase in pH and decrease in PaCO2. With a respiratory rate of 38, the PaO2 is going to be decreased due to the ventilation/perfusion mismatch. When the patient becomes too fatigued, they may go into a state of hypercapnia and acidosis will occur eventually.

17) **Correct answer: A** Cyanide can be found in everyday items such as insulation, furniture coverings and carpets. These items can release cyanide if they catch fire. High temperatures and low oxygen concentrations favor the formation of cyanide gas. Cyanide impedes the aerobic metabolism process during ATP formation in the electron transport chain causing an anaerobic state.

18) **Correct answer: B** With this patient, recall Dalton's Law: as you increase in altitude, the barometric pressure decreases, causes the partial pressure of oxygen to decrease. This means that the available oxygen decreases as we ascend in altitude. A patient's PO2 at sea level on 21% oxygen is 159 mmHg and is cut in half (70 mmHg) at 18,000 ft MSL.

19) **Correct answer: B** Polycythemia is sometimes called erythrocytosis, but the terms are not synonymous because polycythemia refers to any increase in red blood cells, whereas erythrocytosis only refers to a documented increase of red cell

mass. The overproduction of red blood cells may be due to a primary process in the bone marrow (a so-called myeloproliferative syndrome), or it may be a reaction to chronically low oxygen levels.

20) **Correct answer: C** Looking at the patient's ventilation status identifies acute respiratory failure. Any PaCO2 level that is above 50mmHg is an indicator of respiratory failure. In addition, a PO2 of < 60 mmHg is an indication of hypoxic respiratory failure.

21) **Correct answer: A** Histotoxic hypoxia occurs when metabolic disorders or poisoning of the cytochrome oxidase enzyme system results in a cell's inability to use molecular oxygen. Histotoxic hypoxia interferes with the utilization phase of respiration because of metabolic poisoning or dysfunction. Specific causes of Histotoxic hypoxia could include respiratory enzyme poisoning or degradation and the intake of carbon monoxide, cyanide, or alcohol.

22) **Correct answer: D** Remember the concept of absorptive atelectasis. Nitrogen is 78% of atmospheric air. It's very dense and doesn't diffuse in low O2 states (21%). In high concentrations however, it will be displaced by O2. Use the rule of 5 X FiO2 = PO2!

23) **Correct answer: D** Remember, a good way to determine tube depth after watching it go through the cords, is 3 x tube size.

24) **Correct answer: D** Neuromuscular blocking agents, specifically succinylcholine, have a higher incidence than PCN and latex allergies.

25) **Correct answer: D** Although Fentanyl, in high doses (>3mcg/kg), will achieve sedation, Fentanyl's primary use is to blunt the sympathetic response associated with intubation. We want to blunt that huge pain response.

26) **Correct answer: A** Remember that when administering succinylcholine, the properties of the medication can cause a massive release of K+ post 12 hours of burn due to the non-competitive mechanism of the medication. Always choose another form of paralysis in these patients by using a competitive neuromuscular blocking agent like Rocuronium or Vecuronium.

FlightBridgeED, LLC
Chapter 3 | Dominating Transport Ventilation

1) **Correct answer**: Rationale - The biggest aspect to this patient presentation is the obstructive lung disease. When dealing with obstructive lung patients, it's paramount to allow the patient ample time to exhale. The protective aspect of this approach is the low (f). This patient is being ventilated with a (f) of 32. COPD or asthma patients need a slow (f) so as to allow them time to exhale. In addition, the patient has a PEEP of 15 cm H2O. He/she most certainly has a high auto-PEEP and this is just increasing intra-thoracic pressure and reducing chest wall compliance. The Vte has decreased significantly as well. The treatment for this patient is to first disconnect the ventilator from the ETT to allow exhalation. Next, reduce the (f) to 12-14. Lastly, remove the PEEP and set it between 0-3 cm H20. If you notice, the PaO2 is fine, then the patient probably has a low SaO2 because of the poor minute ventilation secondary to the poor compliance, high PEEP, and high (f). Lastly, set the I:E ratio to 1:4 -1:5 for the longer exhalation time. Once you correct those items, the patient's SaO2 will improve.
2) **Correct answer**: Rationale - The big lesson with this presentation is that pediatric patients are often hard to assess. Lung sounds need to be performed very axillary due to the potential for chest sounds echoing. Second, if you see the P_{plat} increase suddenly, this goes for any patient, this is an indication that alveolar pressures have increased and chest wall compliance is poor. In addition, the EtCO2 has gone up significantly as well, telling you

that there is some type of shunt happening. Match that with the mechanism, and you should immediately perform chest decompression on the affected side. If unsure, then perform bilateral decompressions.
3) **Correct answer: A** PIP being elevated with a normal P$_{plat}$ is a direct indication of upper airway involvement, volume, flow, airway constriction, pulmonary toilet, ETT kink, or vent circuit kink! Think above the carina!
4) **Correct answer: Rationale** Remember, volume always equals increased pressure. Look at the IBW and how high the Vt is. It would suggest decreasing Vt to 420-450 and re-evaluate the PIP and P$_{plat}$.
5) **Correct answer: Rationale** This biggest aspect in regards to this patient presentation is the metabolic acidosis and DKA. Make sure you match the patient's spontaneous rate or match their EtCO2 prior to intubation. Any change in PaCO2 will affect pH in the opposite direction. A 10mmHg increase will cause a decrease of 0.08 in pH.
6) **Correct answer: Rationale** The patient's P$_{plat}$ pressure will be your most indicative sign that your patient has a progressing tension pneumothorax. When you see this, never wait to decompress your patient.
7) **Correct answer: C** Pressure control ventilation, although very good for hypoxic patients, or patients with poor chest compliance ("baby lungs"), is based on lung compliance, so you do not have a guaranteed V$_E$. The Vt will change based on changes with chest wall compliance.

8) **Correct answer: D** When administering nitrates of any kind (NTG, nipride, nitroprusside, nitric oxide), the clinician needs to keep in mind that the byproduct of these medications is cyanide, which causes methemoglobinemia. Essentially, the cyanide blocks O2 conversion in the electron transport chain and inhibits aerobic metabolism. The patient develops clinical indications of hypoxia and decreased arterial oxygen saturation, but will have a normal PaO2. Normal methemoglobin levels are 1-2%. When patients have methemoglobin levels that exceed 10%, this will often result in the beginning stages of hypoxia. Treatment for these patients would be discontinuation of the offending agent and IV administration of methylene blue for patients who are symptomatic and have a methemoglobin level >30%.

9) **Correct answer: B** P_{plat} is the most sensitive marker for alveolar health. Trending the P_{plat} during initial ventilator set up and throughout your care is essential to identify high pressure that will damage the lungs, alveoli and cause VLI, inflammatory cascades and barotrauma.

10) **Correct answer: C** SIMV is the most dynamic mode of ventilation and provides three levels of ventilator support. First, it will guarantee a minute ventilation (V_E) for an apneic patient. Second, it will allow the patient to take spontaneous breaths based on the trigger and augment those spontaneous breaths with the addition of pressure support (PS). Third, it will allow the patient to completely control the ventilator if the patient has the necessary respiratory drive.

11) **Correct answer: A** Pressure limited volume control ventilation is the gentlest way to ventilate your patients. Always remember your patients are sick and have "baby" lungs. Pressure modes of ventilation are based on compliance and will only apply a pressure based on that compliance.

12) **Correct answer: C** Airway pressures are the most important parameter to monitor on your ventilated patient. PIP, P$_{plat}$ and static compliance tells you many things as it relates to alveolar health, barotrauma and overall lung health.
13) **Correct answer: C** With any metabolic acidosis, always remember to allow the patient to compensate. If the patient is paralyzed, then match their respiratory rate and EtCO2 reading prior to intubation so as to continue blowing off excess acid (CO2). This will prevent the pH from decreasing. Remember the winter's formula. For every 10mmHg of change in PaCO2, you will have an inverse change in pH by 0.08.
14) **Correct answer: B** When attempting to increase oxygenation in patients that are hypoxic, always increase the FiO2 first and PEEP second. With the answers available, increasing PEEP would be your best choice.
15) **Correct answer: B** When you look at ventilator pressures, always look first at the PIP. This looks at volume, compliance, airway resistance and flow. If this is high, then check your P$_{plat}$. If this reflects low, you know that this elevation in pressure is due to something above the carina. If the PIP is high and you have a P$_{plat}$ that is high as well, remember the elevated P$_{plat}$ is causing the transient pressure change in the upper airways, and the problem is at the alveolar level.
16) **Correct answer: C** Dead space is an aspect that many forget to account for. If not accounted for, you will cause hypoventilation. Remember that for each breath you lose approximately 150mL per breath. Using the 1mL/IBW for your dead space calculation, you will allow for this and increase your minute ventilation (V$_E$) to account for this loss. Understanding that overall V$_E$ is different than alveolar minute ventilation (V$_A$). Accounting for dead

space allows you to identify your desire alveolar minute V$_A$. If you use this equation below, you will account for dead space and maintain eucapnia. – 120mL/kg/min = desired V$_A$.

17) **Correct answer: B** The PaO2 is low on this patient. This problem can be improved by increasing the FiO2 or PEEP. Because the FiO2 is already at 0.6 and the PEEP is only at 5, an increase in the PEEP would be the most preferable choice because this is most likely ARDS. In most patients, increasing the FiO2 would be your first choice. However, remember that increasing FiO2 for long periods leads to the release of free radicals, causes nitrogen washout and atelectasis trauma and will worsen the inflammatory cascade already in full effect from the surgery. A PEEP of 5 is considered physiologic, not therapeutic. You should make the effort to limit the amount of FiO2 that the patient requires to the least amount possible to prevent oxygen toxicity over a period of time.

18) **Correct answer: A** This would be an underlying metabolic acidosis with a mixed disturbance because you have respiratory and kidney involvement showing an acidosis. Your PaCO2 is 70 and HCO3 is 14.

19) **Correct answer: C** Pressure regulated volume control uses volume targeted-pressure limited delivery to achieve Vt. The ventilator is constantly checking compliance and volume to regulate the pressure to achieve the desired Vt. This is very safe, effective and gentle for the patients.

20) **Correct answer: D** The patient is presenting with a probable oxygenation and ventilation failure, but is still maintaining her airway. Anytime we can optimize oxygenation and ventilation without placing an ETT and making the patient ventilator dependent, the patient is going to do better. Using BiPAP will allow you to keep the patient off the ventilator and assist her in improving by using the Bi-level mode of

ventilation. Remember, your IPAP is your minute ventilation (V_E) and the ePAP is the oxygenation. Using a starting iPAP of 10 and ePAP of 5 will give you a good staring point and can monitor her progress. If you feel like this is more of an oxygenation problem, move the iPAP to 12 and ePAP to 7. Increases should occur together by 2-3 cmH20. If you feel this is more of a ventilation failure, move the iPAP to 12 and the ePAP down to 3. This allows for a greater gradient for her to exhale over.

21) **Correct answer: D** When treating a patient with any obstructive lung disease, remember that the number one objective is to allow the patient optimal time to exhale. In the patient presentation, using an I:E ratio of 1:4 is the best option. This approach, along with lowering the patient's (f) will allow the patient optimal time to blow off the retained $PaCO2$.

22) **Correct answer: D** In the scenario, the mechanism and initial assessment should give you a high index of suspicion that this patient has a probable pneumothorax and it's likely to progress to a tension pneumothorax. Taking the patient off the ventilator and bagging the patient is not going to solve the underlying problem. It's a late sign to have BVM compliance diminish to the point of identifying a tension. The P_{plat} is going to be the most sensitive indication of impending problems at the alveolar level and tell you that the simple pneumothorax you identified is now a tension. Immediate chest decompression on the effect side or bilaterally is warranted. This is a life threat and needs to be an immediate action by the clinician.

23) **Correct answer: C** When monitoring a patient on volume control ventilation, consistent monitoring of the patient's pressures are essential. Specific attention should be focused on the P_{plat}. The PIP and P_{plat} are specific indicators of airway health.

Always remember that your PIP is an indication of upper airway health and the P$_{plat}$ is an indication of lower airway (alveolar health). Static compliance is an indication of overall chest/lung compliance and should be between 50-70 cmH20.

When you start to see pressures that exceed this and become greater than 100 cmH20, the patient has excessive pressures and the lung/chest wall compliance is starting to hinder normal lung function.

24) **Correct answer: D** Using SIMV has become the primary mode of ventilation when dealing with patients that are ventilator dependent. Research has shown that assist control causes respiratory muscle atrophy and severely hinders patients being weaned off the ventilator. SIMV is now used around the country for a primary mode because it always allows the patient the ability to take some type of spontaneous breath. With the addition of pressure support (PS), the patient is able to take an augmented breath and it reduces the work of breathing. The objective is to allow some patient induced respiratory effort, without causing muscle fatigue. It's important to establish a PS reading that is at least 5 cm H20 greater than your current PEEP. So if your PEEP is set at 5 cm H20, then set your PS at a minimum of 10 cm H20. This helps eliminate dead space that is currently in the ETT and ventilator circuit. You then want to monitor those spontaneous breaths. You don't want the patients spontaneous breaths to exceed 75% of your set Vt. So if your Vt is set at 400 mL, your patient's spontaneous breath shouldn't exceed 300 mL. If this happens, treat the patient with an analgesic medication and sedation.

25) **Correct answer: C** When establishing Pressure Control Ventilation (PCV), your starting inspiratory pressure (Pinsp) is the sum of the current Peak Inspiratory Pressure (PIP) and PEEP. This is the maximum pressure you may have to overcome in

the patient's airway. However, this is a starting pressure and the clinician will need to immediately identify based on the exhaled tidal volume (Vte) if this is too little or greater than the desire ideal body weight calculated Vt.

Chapter 4 | Flight Physiology

1) **Correct answer: B** In these types of questions, always take the least amount of time if it's above 30,000 ft MSL.
2) **Correct answer: C** Barotitis media will show itself during descent. During the ascent phase of flight, the gas will expand in the ear. Due to the plugged ear, or respiratory infection, the gas will be trapped and cause pain on descent.
3) **Correct answer: A** Think of how your tires on your car expand in the summer and decrease in size during the winter months. As you increase the temperature, the air in an enclosed space will expand. You can also relate this to your cascade O2 cylinder. As the temperature increases throughout the day, the amount of O2 pressure in the tank will increase proportionally.
4) **Correct answer: C** Barodentalgia will worsen on ascent. As you ascend, you will have a dull or severe pain depending on if it's secondary to a filling (severe) or an abscess (dull) pain and the pressure will increase in the tooth. This is the concept of Boyle's Law.
5) **Correct answer: D** Dalton's law or (Dalton's gang) essentially states that as we ascend in altitude, the concentration of O2 remains the same. However, because of the decreased barometric pressure, the partial pressure (PO2) of oxygen decreases as the altitude increases. So, in the simplest terms, imagine if you had a zip lock bag filled with oxygen molecules. At sea level, the oxygen molecules would have a greater pressure exerted against them (760 torr). At 40,000ft, the same concentration of

oxygen would have 162 torr of pressure exerted against the oxygen molecules, thus the partial pressure becomes very low. Now, the same amount of oxygen at sea level (159 PO2) is now only 34 PO2, at 40,000ft. See example below.
At sea level: 760torr X .21 = 159 PO2
40,000ft: 162torr x .21 = 34 PO2

6) **Correct answer: C** Remember, these questions can be tricky. We are sitting currently at 1 ATM. For every 33ft the diver descends, he is accounting for another ATM. So, if he is at 1 ATM, and he has descended 99ft, he is at 4 ATMs.

7) **Correct answer: C** Giving high concentrations of O2 is affecting Henry's law and the solubility of oxygen diffusion. Graham's law affects the active process of diffusion, which is moving from higher concentration to lower concentration. Henry's law is affecting the concentration, the solubility and the pressure that oxygen molecules need to be placed under to diffuse more rapidly into a solution (blood). ***Remember the rule of FiO2 X 5 = Potential PO2***

8) **Correct answer: D** When answering this question, any time you have a rapid decompression you cut your time of useful consciousness in half. Always choose the shortest time frame when answering this question.

9) **Correct answer: D** As we ascend in altitude the barometric pressure decreases. This allows more gas to occupy a space. Boyle's law states, as we increase in altitude the volume increase as barometric pressure decreases.

10) **Correct answer: A** Anytime you see a question related to ascent and flight, remember Boyle's law is the gas law that drives increased pressure with the decrease in barometric pressure in ascent.

11) **Correct answer: B** When thinking about this gas law always think about a carbonated drink. The drink, when unopened, has a higher amount of pressure above the solution. When you open the drink the pressure above the fluid immediately equalizes with the atmosphere, becoming lower than the pressure of the gas dissolved in the beverage. Additionally, we need to understand that this is our most important gas law as it relates to oxygenation. We can apply it by doing three things. First, increase the concentration. By increasing FiO2 to 100% you in-turn start driving up the PO2. Next, we need to increase the surface area by adding PEEP. If we increase the alveolar membrane's size, we then have more area for gas exchange. Last, we put the solution under pressure. By adding positive pressure via a BVM or the ventilator, we then push those increased O2 molecules through the solution (blood).

12) **Correct answer: C** At sea level, the dissolved gases in the blood and tissues are in proportion to the partial pressures of the gases in the person's lungs at the surface. As the diver descends underwater, the ambient pressure increases, and therefore the pressure of the gas inside the lungs increases correspondingly. Because the partial pressures of the gases in the lungs are now greater than the dissolved partial pressures of these gases in the blood and tissues, gas molecules begin to move from the lungs into the blood and tissues. Eventually, the concentration of the dissolved gases in the blood and tissues will be proportional to the partial pressures in the breathing gas (i.e., a state of equilibrium). However, if the diver resurfaces too quickly and as the pressure decreases as he/she comes to the surface, the

excess nitrogen can't be dissolved in the lungs quick enough causing decompression sickness, thus causing the possibility of the bends, creeps, chokes and staggers.

13) **Correct answer: C** Charles law states that a change in temperature will cause a change in volume assuming that the pressure remains constant. If you were to let a balloon increase in altitude, that balloon would have a decrease in volume as temperature decreases. For every 1000' of increase in altitude you decrease in temperature 2° C.

14) **Correct answer: A** If you were to let a balloon increase in altitude, that balloon would have a decrease in volume as temperature decreased. For every 1000' of increase in altitude you decrease in temperature 2° C.

15) **Correct answer: C** Because of the aspects of Boyles' law, the ever changing altitude and pressures, drip rates can be difficult to maintain. The best option in flight is to place fluids on a pressure bag and then titrate the drip rate under pressure. This pressure will overcome any pressure increases associated with altitude differences and Boyles' Law.

FlightBridgeED, LLC
Chapter 5 | Environmental Emergencies

1) **Correct answer: C** All of the above are important aspects of how we compensate. However, glycogen stores will limit one's ability to shiver and produce heat.
2) **Correct answer: B** With temperatures below $30°$ C, the medication pharmacodynamics mechanism of action will not work, thus causing the medication to build up in the system.
3) **Correct answer: Rationale** This is a tough patient. This patient is suffering from multiple problems. His labs are showing severe dehydration with hyponatremia and hypokalemia from the tap water feedings and the hot apartment. Controlling the airway and slowing the seizure activity should be your first priority. Correcting the blood sugar would be next. The patient's serum osmolality is elevated signaling a shift to the extravascular spaces. This is causing cerebral swelling and is progressing his neurological dysfunction. Treating the hyponatremia needs to be your next treatment using a 3% saline or other hypertonic fluid; however this needs to happen very slowly. Raising Na+ levels too quickly will lead to central pontine myelinosis. Hyponatremia should be corrected at a rate of no more than 8-10 mmol/L of sodium per day. The patient already has cerebral edema caused by the hypovolemia and hyponatremia. Don't make it worse.
4) **Correct answer: A** Rewarming needs to take place in the most physiologic manner possible. Active external would take place by a heater source; passive external would be removing wet cloths and using the patients own body to warm itself via blankets. Active internal rewarming would include

humidified O2 and warm IV fluids ECMO, gastric lavage, and intubation.
5) **Correct answer: C** Cimetadine is an H2 blocker used to treat ulcers. In the hyperthermic patient it is used to prevent ulcers due to the stress response. The body will try to increase glucose production by releasing cortisol. This release of cortisol causes a reduction of PGE production, which slows GI mucous synthesis.
6) **Correct answer: B** All of the answers are correct except for "oxygen supply exceeds demand". In the hyperthermic patient there will be a high demand and low supply. We need to optimize oxygenation through all means necessary.
7) **Correct answer: C** The earliest lab value that identifies muscle damage and release of myoglobin is going to be your CK. Creatine kinase is an enzyme that is present in all the muscles of the body and is a catalyst in the energy conversion process. Creatine kinase used in the body are of two types - for the muscles and for the brain.
8) **Correct answer: C** Rhabdomyolysis occurs when damaged skeletal muscle (myoglobin) tissue breaks down causing damage to the kidneys. Myoglobin is the oxygen carrier for the muscle tissue. Very similar to hemoglobin. However, it's very toxic when released outside of muscle tissue. Hyperthermia and prolonged seizure activity can both lead to the development. The elevated CK is the first indicator, along with increases in BUN and Cr, indicating kidney damage. Immediate fluid resuscitation with a targeted urine output of 100mL/hr and the administration of a NaHCO3 drip to alkalinize the urine, along with either Mannitol or Lasix to pull the fluid off, is the standard treatment.

9) **Correct answer: B** When malignant hyperthermia manifests, it's usually in response to the administration of succinylcholine. Because of the depolarizing aspects of the medication, and the fasciculations, massive calcium release can occur. This causes a systemic muscle firing throughout the body and the muscle rigidity generates excessive heat. This causes an immediate rise in body temperature.

10) **Correct answer: D** When malignant hyperthermia manifests, it's usually in response to the administration of succinylcholine. Initial s/s will be: masseter spasms and/or trismus, despite the paralytic administration, a rapidly increasing EtCO2, tachycardia, and hypertension. The treatment is to administer Dantrolene Sodium 2.5 mg/kg until s/s stop and aggressive cooling measures.

11) **Correct answer: A** When dealing with drowning, and understanding the difference with fresh water and salt water drowning, it's important to realize that although they may seem similar, fresh water drowning causes systemic washout of the surfactant, which is important for alveolar health. Without it, atelectasis trauma and collapse will ensue. With salt water drowning, the salt causes a hyperosmolar shift and third spacing of blood and plasma into the pulmonary spaces. This will need to be treated with your ventilator, very similar to how we treat patients with ARDS or pneumonia. Lower Vt, higher f, and higher PEEP.

Chapter 6 | Hematology & Electrolytes

1) **Correct answer: C** Although treatment for correction of DIC is intense and controversial, the main focus should always be treating the underlying problem. If the patient is suffering from a massive head injury, do what is necessary to correct the problem and the DIC will ultimately correct.
2) **Correct answer: C** The H&H will normally increase by 1 & 3 with each unit of PRBCs. Also, remember that the Hct is approximately 3 times that of the Hgb.
3) **Correct answer: B** Fever and diaphoresis leads to free water loss through the skin leading to a state of hypernatremia. Diarrhea and vomiting both lead to Na+ and water loss. Loop diuretics usually result in hyponatremia due to hypovolemia. SIADH leads to hyponatremia due to increased water reabsorption that occurs in the renal tubules.
4) **Correct answer: C** Normal magnesium levels are 1.5-2.5 mEq/L. Hypermagnesemia manifestations result from depressed neuromuscular transmission. Absence of reflexes reflect a magnesium level around 7 mEq/L. Hypotension is also a manifestation.
5) **Correct answer: C** Hypokalemia results in inverted T waves, ST segment depression, and prominent U waves.
6) **Correct answer: B** Hypoparathyroidism causes the body to secrete low levels of parathyroid hormone. This hormone maintains and regulates calcium and phosphorus. These findings are indicative of a decrease in serum calcium. This would cause an increased phosphorus level as well, because

calcium and phosphorus have an inverse relationship.

7) **Correct answer: B** Dehydration is the most common cause of an increased hematocrit. As the volume of fluid in the blood drops, the RBCs per volume of fluid rise. The Na+ levels also rise due to the loss of fluid or volume during a state of dehydration. Remember, it's a concentration based on the fluid.

8) **Correct answer: A** Lasix can result in a state of hyponatremia. Signs of hyponatremia include: apprehension, abdominal cramps, diarrhea and convulsions. Oliguria and sticky mucous membranes are indicative of hypernatremia. Increases in urine specific gravity occur in states of dehydration or SIADH.

9) **Correct answer: C** DIC occurs from over stimulation of the clotting cascade resulting in clots being formed in the body's small blood vessels. Although these patients will bleed due to the excessive clotting using up all the body's platelets and clotting factors, the primary problem is with clotting.

10) **Correct answer: B** Citrate is used for anticoagulation in PRBCs. Rapid administration of PRBCs can lead to an accumulation of citrate. Normally, the liver metabolizes citrate quickly, but in some instances, toxicity can occur. This normally results in patients with liver dysfunction or neonates with immature liver function. It can result in hypocalcemia and hypomagnesaemia when the citrate binds with calcium and magnesium.

11) **Correct answer: A** In citrate toxicity, the citrate binds with calcium and magnesium and causes hypocalcemia and hypomagnesaemia. These patients will present with signs of hypocalcemia, which needs to be restored. Remember, Ca++ is

essential for vascular tone and inotropic aspects on the heart.

12) **Correct answer: C** PRBCs are high in potassium due to hemolysis. Signs of hyperkalemia on the ECG include tall, peaked T waves and QRS complex widening.

13) **Correct answer: D** The creatinine clearance directly reflects the GFR. It is an evaluation of the ability of the kidneys to filter waste products, such as creatinine.

14) **Correct answer: B** DIC is a coagulopathy that will consume all platelets and clotting factors. All clotting studies are prolonged. The primary treatment for DIC is resolution of the offending agent.

15) **Correct answer: B** If you are trying to identify the patient's metabolic disorder and you don't have an ABG to reference, the quickest calculation to identify a metabolic acidosis is via an anion gap. You can calculate an uncorrected anion gap or a corrected anion gap. See below:
Uncorrected = Na+ - (Cl + HCO3) *If > 12 you have a metabolic acidosis*.
Corrected = Na+ - (Cl + HCO3) + K+ *If > 20 you have a metabolic acidosis (Most accurate)*

16) **Correct answer: A** Dehydration causes an excessive loss of total body water leading to a state of hypernatremia. Hypernatremia can cause lethargy, weakness, irritability, neuromuscular excitability and edema. If left untreated, it can lead to seizures or coma.

17) **Correct answer: C** Hypocalcemia can cause numbness and tingling in the perioral area, muscle cramps/spasms and irritability/fatigue. Two common tests for hypocalcemia include Chvostek's sign and Trousseau's sign.

FlightBridgeED, LLC
Chapter 7 | CAMTS

1) **Correct answer: C** 12 o'clock will always be the first meeting point in any emergency situation. If that is not available, then move to 3 o'clock and so on. Stay away from any moving parts and don't exit until the rotor has stopped.
2) **Correct answer: B** Always turn the RPM's down, then cut the fuel, then the power, with your O2 being last!!
3) **Correct answer: D** Always remember... VFR=VMC. For IFR flight, you need to file a flight plan and have an IFR equipped aircraft, pilot and GPS approach, certified LZ, or airport.
4) **Correct answer: D** Always know the location of your aircrafts ELT. Beware that it may or may not activate at 4 G's. Always attempt to access and remove it in the case of a crash landing if safe to do so.
5) **Correct answer: A** Always be responsible for understanding weather minimums and current weather conditions. It's just as much your responsibility as it is the pilots. You owe it to your family!
6) **Correct answer: B** This question is a knowledge recall question. 1/4" is the correct response to allow the proper insulation and fit between you and your flight suit.
7) **Correct answer: A** This is also a recall type question. Day-time local minimums are 800' and 2 miles. The old 8th edition standards were 500' and 1 mile. Most companies have exceeded those standards and have adopted the 800' and 2. When CAMTS came out with the 9th edition, they increased these minimums as well.

8) **Correct answer: D** Although a company can exceed the CAMTS recommendations and require more, the CAMTS standard is 5 live or HPS intubations.
9) **Correct answer: A** This is a maximum time of response only. Obviously we need to respond as quickly as safely possible.
10) **Correct answer: A** All answers except for (A) are correct. An ATP certificate is for an aircraft mechanic only. Pilots do not need to have or maintain this certification.
11) **Correct answer: C** These questions are standard CAMTS questions. It takes 4 G's to activate the ELT. You should always know where the ELT is located and how to manually activate it.
12) **Correct answer: D** Although the pilot is the person in command of the aircraft and makes weather decisions, any crewmember on the aircraft can say "no" It take 3 to go and 1 to say no.
13) **Correct answer: D** All critical phases of flight.
14) **Correct answer: B** The correct answer is to identify another route that is safe and allows you to get the patient to the definitive facility. Safety is paramount and attempting to drive through the flooded roadway would put the entire crew and patient is an unsafe situation. Calling for back up, although a good choice, would not get you out of the unsafe situation and allow the patient the best chance to arrive safely at the receiving destination.
15) **Correct answer: C** The best choice in this scenario is to get yourself and your patient out of danger. If you have the option to move to a curb or sidewalk out of the roadway that would always be the safest option. Although we're taught to move to the 12 or 3 O'clock location if you're in an aircraft accident, roadway accidents offer extra dangers. The 12 or 3 O'clock location would potentially place you in the road

way and in further danger. Staying in the ambulance would also pose further danger for you and your patient by placing you in a potential situation of being hit by another vehicle.

16) **Correct answer: B**

17) **Correct answer: B** The simplex system is being used in this scenario. The simplex system uses old, simple technology that has a single channel for transmit and receive and is considered VHF. The signal travels in one direction only. These systems however have limited range due to its single channel capability and the inability to use a repeater for longer-range communications.

Chapter 8 | Cardiac Physiology

1) **Correct answer: C** 10% of the population is LAD dominant. This means that these patients will have inferior wall involvement with associated lateral wall infarcts. The left circumflex feeds the inferior wall instead of the right coronary artery.
2) **Correct answer: A** Augmentation of the left ventricle revolves around allowing the ventricle to fill properly. Often, treatment of HTN (ACE Inhibitors and Beta Blockers) are first line treatments, along with digoxin for inotropic augmentation and contractility.
3) **Correct answer: B** Sgarbossa criteria is evident due to positive concordance seen in V1 along with 5mm elevation seen in Lead II and III. This would be highly suspicious for an ACS event and should be treated as such!!!
4) **Correct answer: C** In the patient presenting with cardiogenic shock, it is often easy to diagnose based on presentation. However, understanding lab values and the use of BNP as a guide to CHF diagnosis is essential in the critical care arena. BNP is an enzyme released due to overstretch of the ventricles.
5) **Correct answer: C** Nitroglycerin is a potent vasodilator and as such will decrease preload and afterload. This is a good thing in most cases of MI. However, inferior wall MI's are associated with RVI (right ventricular infarction) 50% of the time. RVI will cause a massive container failure and a corresponding huge decrease in preload!

6) **Correct answer: C** With any patient suffering from an inferior MI, always remember that 50% of all inferior MI's have an associated right ventricular infarction. This will lead to severe preload failure. In any inferior wall MI, take a few seconds and check for a right-sided MI by doing a right sided 12-lead using V4R. If positive, these patients need fluid, fluid, and more fluid. Optimize preload and then you can start giving small doses of Nitroglycerin. If available, start a nitro drip instead of using nitro sprays.

7) **Correct answer: A** When looking at an inferior wall MI, think about which artery is feeding this area. The right anterior descending artery feeds the inferior and posterior walls. Posterior wall MI's are most often associated with inferior MI's. If you see inferior wall involvement in leads II, III, and AVF, and depression in V1-V4, this is diagnostic for a posterior MI. You can also do a posterior 12-lead by doing V7-V12, but is not often done in the field do to the inferior involvement. Just treat the inferior wall MI and you will treat the posterior automatically.

8) **Correct answer: B** This diagnostic test is sometimes difficult to see. Always match this with the presentation and history of the present illness. Remember: **S1, Q3, T3 [s wave in lead 1, pathological Q wave in lead III, inverted T wave in lead III]**.

9) **Correct answer: D** Neo-synephrine is an excellent medication to use in the septic shock or neurogenic shock patient. It has potent alpha effects without causing an increase in heart rate and O2 demand.

10) **Correct answer: A** Sgarbossa criteria is a diagnostic test that awards a point system to LBBB or RBBB. In the past, LBBB were hard to identify in association with ACS. Often, patients were not

reperfused quickly enough. Mortality for LBBB in conjunction with ACS is very high. Sgarbossa devised a point system that looks at ST segment elevation = or > 1 mm that is concordant with the QRS complex, along with ST elevation of 5mm or greater in any lead that is discordant to the QRS complex. If the LBBB is identified to have discordant T waves to the QRS deflection, then this is a normal finding and doesn't indicate an associated MI with the LBBB. Concordant T waves mean the deflection of the T wave is going in the same direction as the QRS complex. A discordant T waves mean the deflection of the T wave is going opposite of the QRS complex.

11) **Correct answer: B** It is seen in cardiac tamponade and severe pericardial effusion and is thought to be related to changes in the ventricular electrical axis due to fluid in the pericardium, as the heart essentially wobbles in the fluid filled pericardial sac. This phenomenon causes alternation of QRS complex amplitude or axis between beats, and a possible wandering base line.

12) **Correct answer: B** The gas law that affects this patient and increases the shock state regarding hypoxic hypoxia is Dalton's law. Dalton's law would cause the partial pressure of O2 to decrease. Think of an increase in altitude will cause a decrease in barometric pressure and thus cause a reduction in available O2.

13) **Correct answer: D** Mitral regurgitation following an inferior MI is a common finding. The inferior MI can cause ischemia to the posterior leaflet of the mitral valve causing the regurgitation. This is the classic finding of a holosystolic murmur radiating to the

axilla as well. Mitral regurgitation causes pulmonary edema due to the backward flow of the right ventricle.

14) **Correct answer: C** Blood pressure is a component of SVR and afterload. In order to reduce this patient's BP, you need to reduce the afterload. Arterial vasodilators (such as hydralazine) reduce the afterload.

15) **Correct answer: B** In sepsis and early septic shock, the cardiac output and contractility are increased as well as the heart rate. Preload and afterload are decreased due to the vasodilation that takes place during sepsis.

16) **Correct answer: C** Over-sensing occurs when the pacemaker senses impulses besides what is intended and is inhibited by this.

17) **Correct answer: B** A LBBB will cause widened QRS complexes greater than 0.12 seconds and positive R waves in leads V5 and V6. It will also cause negative QS wave in V1. LBBB will also cause a paradoxical splitting of S2, which causes the split on expiration but not on inspiration. It is considered paradoxical because it is opposite of a normal split S2, which is split on inspiration but not on expiration.

18) **Correct answer: B** Coronary artery perfusion is dependent on end diastolic pressures. Think about how an IABP works. You are optimizing coronary artery perfusion by reducing afterload and perfusing the coronary arteries during the diastolic phase.

19) **Correct answer: C** Leads II, III, and aVF view the inferior wall of the left ventricle. This is supplied by the right coronary artery (RCA). The RCA supplies the AV node in 90% of the population. Occlusion of the RCA causes changes such as first- and second-degree AV block and Mobitz type I.

20) **Correct answer: A** Chronic atrial fibrillation will cause blood to stay within the atria causing wall thrombi. These thrombi may cause secondary emboli throughout the body. About 30% of all strokes are estimated to be the result of atrial fibrillation. The prophylactic administration of warfarin prevents the development of these thrombi in the atria.

21) **Correct answer: C** When dealing with patients suffering from an anterior wall MI, the artery that supplies this area is the left main coronary artery. You have to remember that the mitral valve is supplying blood into the left ventricle and as such is a very high-pressure valve. This valve is controlled by small leaflets that open and close it. When an MI is present in that area (anterior wall), it often causes damage or complete detachment from the mitral valve causing mitral valve regurgitation/insufficiency. Due to this phenomenon, you will have extreme backflow of blood into the lungs and flash pulmonary edema. The patient's airway needs to be stabilized immediately by endotracheal intubation. In addition, the patient will need emergent surgical repair or replacement of the mitral valve along with other cardiac support measures including IABP and Impella devices.

22) **Correct answer: C** Treatment goals for patient's suffering from left ventricular failure is aimed at optimizing stroke volume, preload, afterload, and contractility. Over diuresis may result in an abnormal reduction in preload that causes an under stretch of the left ventricle and decreased contractility. Fluid boluses are often given to restore adequate circulating blood volume and to optimize preload, stroke volume and cardiac output. In patients presenting in this manner, it is most appropriate to

use venous vasodilators, because of how easy they are to titrate, in hopes to reduce preload in a hemodynamically unstable patient. Even though there was a decrease in PCWP from 16 mmHg to 8 mmHg, patients suffering from left ventricular failure often need a wedge pressure that is higher to allow for optimal stretch especially in patients with a diseased heart with a larger ventricular diameter.

23) **Correct answer: B** Blocking only the beta-receptors during cocaine overdose results in increasing HTN, reduction in coronary blood flow, left ventricular function and cardiac output. This results in a reduction in tissue perfusion because the alpha-adrenergic system is left unopposed. Appropriate antihypertensive medications to use during cocaine overdose include vasodilators such as NTG, diuretics, and alpha-blockers.

24) **Correct answer: C** ACE inhibitors block the stimulation of the RAA system. When the RAA system is stimulated by hypo-perfusion of the kidney, it causes vasoconstriction and sodium and water retention. Stimulation of the RAA system would lead to further deterioration in a heart failure patient.

25) **Correct answer: B** You know this patient has a decrease in contractility so the only way to improve these symptoms is to increase his contractility with an inotropic agent such as dobutamine. Failure of the heart has caused the fluid to back up into the lungs causing the patient's findings of crackles on auscultation. Additional fluid will not improve this patient's symptoms and can make them worse. Diuretics, such as Lasix, will not increase cardiac output and by decreasing preload, could potentially make this worse. There is no indication of a bleeding or clotting problem presently, so FFP would not be indicated.

26) **Correct answer: A** Calcium is the antagonist to hypermagnesemia. The patient is exhibiting signs of hypermagnesemia due to the hypotension, hyporeflexia, and respiratory depression. The drip should be stopped and calcium chloride administered IV to present an imminent arrest.

FlightBridgeED, LLC
Chapter 9 | Hemodynamic monitoring

1) **Correct answer: Rationale** When looking at this scenario, be careful not to get sucked into the wordy explanation. First, look at the HR (58); this should immediately make you concerned with why your patient isn't compensating with some type of tachycardia. Second, your patient is hypotensive as well and would make you think decompensated shock. Next look at the hemodynamic numbers. Your patient has a low CVP, which means that preload is low; the PCWP is also low which is an indication of left sided preload. Then look at your cardiac output, which is indicated by a hyperdynamic cardiac index (CI) of 6.4. Last, your SVR is also very low, which should clue you into some type of distributive shock. Match that with your presentation and this should give you the diagnosis of neurogenic shock.

2) **Correct answer: A** These are just simple hemodynamic parameters. Your CVP is low indicating some type of preload problem. Next look at your CI, which is also low, telling you that cardiac output is low. Next, look at the PA S/D pressures. These are also low, as well as your PCWP, telling you that left sided preload is low as well. Now you've identified that your right and left sided preload are both low with a low cardiac output. Last, look at your SVR, which is hyperdynamic. So, there is vasoconstriction in an attempt to increase cardiac output. You should be looking at simple hypovolemia. Left systolic dysfunction is wrong because you would see high PA S/D and PCWP, which you don't have. Neurogenic shock is wrong because you would see a hyperdynamic cardiac index. Last, sepsis is wrong because you would see

a low SVR as well as other low hemodynamic parameters. So your answer is hypovolemia.

3) **Correct answer: B** Your CVP is high. This indicates higher pressures down stream or in the right ventricle. Next, your CI is low and shows a poor cardiac output. Next your PA S/D pressures are very high. This should tell you that your left heart has a problem or has backpressure. Next, your PCWP is high, telling you that your left atrial pressures are high. Remember, your PCWP is an indication of left sided preload. Last, your SVR is very hyperdynamic at 2100. This should tell you that the patient is attempting to constrict in order to increase cardiac output and overall stroke volume. This all should lead you to look at left systolic dysfunction as your diagnosis.

4) **Correct answer: C** Your preload is low as indicated by the low CVP. Next, look at your cardiac output, which is indicated by a hyperdynamic CI. Next, identify your PA S/D pressures. This tells you end left diastolic pressures. A pressure of 30/14 is a little high but not horribly high. Next, your PCWP is only 6, telling you that left sided preload is low. Last, your SVR is low as well, so there is no compensation happening. This should look similar to the first question. You should identify a diagnosis of neurogenic shock.

5) **Correct answer: D** Your preload is low as indicated by the CVP of only 1. Next, look at your cardiac output that's indicated by a low CI of 1.6. Next, your PA S/D is low as well. Remember, your PA is looking at your left end diastolic pressure. This shows that your left ventricle is not able to sufficiently provide enough stroke volume. In addition, your PCWP is low as well and matches your low PA pressures. Last, your SVR is only 300. There is no constriction and no compensation. I'll give you a hint. Sepsis or septic shock is the only

thing that will show you low hemodynamic numbers in all categories. Your diagnosis is septic shock.

6) **Correct answer: B** When transferring a patient with a PA catheter, always verify placement and be diligent about monitoring your waveforms. If you ever see the waveform change from a PA waveform to the waveform exhibiting a large notch on the left side of the waveform, the catheter has migrated back into the right ventricle. This is very important to identify quickly and your treatment should be to pull the catheter back into the right atrium. Never advance it forward.

7) **Correct answer: C** If you see your waveform change from a nice PA waveform showing the dicrotic notch on the right side to the low amplitude waveform described in this scenario, your catheter has migrated into the wedge position. This is okay for short periods and only while attempting to measure your PCWP; however, in this case, pulling the catheter back, after making sure your balloon is deflated, into the pulmonary artery is the best treatment approach. If in doubt, pull it all the way back into the right atrium giving you the CVP waveform.

8) **Correct answer: CVP** This is a CVP waveform. It's on the higher end of normal at 11 mmHg. Remember, goal related treatment is aimed at raising the CVP higher so as to guide fluid replacement in sepsis and septic shock. You may also see higher CVP pressures in RVI, left ventricular dysfunction and fluid overload.

9) **Correct answer: RV-PA** This is a RV waveform progressing into a PA waveform. Remember the anacrotic notch is sometimes non-visible. Then we see it going into a PA waveform, however, the PA waveform is over-dampened. That means a sharp down stroke, but no bounces, then back to the waveform. The system is too stiff (not

dynamic enough), meaning there is increased resistance or blockage in the system.
10) **Correct answer: PA** This is a PA waveform. Remember the dicrotic notch is on the right side of the waveform. This PA waveform however is over-dampened. That means a sharp down stroke, but no bounces, then back to the waveform. The system is too stiff (not dynamic enough), meaning there is increased resistance or blockage in the system.
11) **Correct answer: CVP-RV** This is a classic CVP to RV waveform. Again, see that the RV waveform has no anacrotic notch. It looks very much like VT. You can see however that the CVP is higher than normal leading you to suspect some type of overload state; RVI, left systolic dysfunction, or fluid overload. Identifying the other hemodynamic parameters would give you the finished diagnosis.
12) **Correct answer: D** PCWP is a direct marker of left atrial pressure and also indirect marker of left end diastolic pressure. It's measured by wedging the PA catheter in the pulmonary artery. Always think of it as reflective of left sided preload status.
13) **Correct answer: D** You are wedging the PA catheter to get a measurement of the left atrial pressure. When you see a V on the waveform while performing the wedge, it shows left atrial filling against a closed mitral valve and thus shows mitral valve disease/regurgitation.
14) **Correct answer: B** When assessing your A-line, you are looking for the dicrotic notch. This is indicative of pulmonic valve closure while using the swan, and aortic valve closure while using the A-line during IABP therapy. The A-line will be used for secondary timing on your balloon pump (IABP).
15) **Correct answer: B** Don't forget that CVP and RAP are looking at the same things. They both reflect preload. Most often the question will just use CVP. You can always identify volume status by

looking at the CVP and titrating your treatment based on those numbers. Standard CVP/RAP readings will be 2-6mmHg.

16) **Correct answer: B** Anytime you see a low CVP always think preload issues. You can also see the cardiac index is low with an associated high SVR which should make you think volume.

17) **Correct answer: C** When you see hemodynamic parameters that are low across the board with a normal or high CI that should lead you to think vasogenic shock. With the associated history of trauma, this would be a classic neurogenic shock.

18) **Correct answer: A** Systolic BP 80mmHg, CI 1.8L/min, and PCWP 30mmHg is showing you that there is a high afterload pressure reflective of the PCWP of 30mmHg. This is showing that left atrial and left end diastolic pressures are high with an associated low systolic pressure.

19) **Correct answer: D** This presentation shows the patient is suffering from a restrictive cardiomyopathy. The walls of the left ventricle are rigid. This does not allow the walls of the ventricle to stretch (Starlings law), thus causing reduced CO, poor ventricular emptying and CHF. Treatment should focus on left ventricular clearing and optimization of cardiac output by increasing contractility.

20) **Correct answer: C** When looking at your hemodynamic parameters, always start with your CVP and ask yourself, is this person fluid depleted or fluid overloaded? If the CVP is low then it's some type of hypovolemia or vasogenic shock. If you have a high CVP then you know they are overloaded. Next look at your PCWP. Remember the wedge pressure is a direct indication of left atrial pressures and will tell you end diastolic pressures or left sided preload. This patient also has an associated low CI that is reflective of a poor cardiac output. Put

all these parameters together and you should come up with cardiogenic shock.

21) **Correct answer: B** With this patient you should have identified that all hemodynamic parameters are low. The only presentation that would show these parameters is septic shock. Start with your CVP always and work from right to left. Your CVP is low so that should make you think "dry". Next, look at your CI. It is also low showing you that CO is diminished. PCWP is your next value. It is also low and will most often follow what the CVP is (only exception is right heart failure). Next, your SVR is also low showing you that the patient can't compensate any longer and needs vasopressor augmentation.

22) **Correct answer: C** Normal SVR is 800-1200 dyne-sec/cm. This measurement is a recall type question. SVR is measured by the following formula:
$$\frac{80 * (MAP-CVP)}{CO}$$

23) **Correct answer: A** Stroke Volume (SV) = End Diastolic Volume – End Systolic Volume

24) **Correct answer: C** The formula for determining MAP is: [SBP + (2 x Diastolic) / 3]

25) **Correct answer: B** Having a good understanding of what your CVP pressure will tell you is essential in providing good patient care. Remember, your CVP will tell you if your patient is volume depleted or volume overloaded. It's that simple. You can use the CVP to guide fluid resuscitation in your sepsis patients by maintaining a CVP of 8-12mmHg or a CVP of 12-15mmHg with patients who suffer from chronic hypertension or left ventricular hypertrophy.

26) **Correct answer: D** The SVO2 is the most accurate way to determine tissue oxygenation and is used in the ICU setting to trend and determine central venous tissue oxygenation. We use this to

determine supply versus demand. The goal is to maintain a level > 70%.

27) **Correct answer: C** The normal range for PCWP is 8-12mmHg. PCWP is a direct reflection of left atrial diastolic pressure as well as left ventricular end diastolic pressure and tells you the status of left sided preload as well as afterload status.

28) **Correct answer: B** When attempting to wedge the PA catheter, always remember to use the syringe that came with the PA catheter and only fill the balloon to 1.5 mL or until you have wedged. Never exceed 1.5mL.

29) **Correct answer: D** Normal PA pressures are: Systolic = 20-30mmHg - Diastolic = 10-15mmHg.

30) **Correct answer: D** Out of all of the answers, the hemodynamic parameters of PAP 48/26 and PCWP 20 are both high and should tell you the patient is overloaded and lead you to diagnose left ventricular failure.

31) **Correct answer: B** Optimal PCWP is approximately 18mmHg, although it varies from patient to patient. Choosing a PCWP of 18mmHg in this patient optimizes their CI, BP, and urine output.

32) **Correct answer: B** A pulmonary embolus leads to pulmonary hypertension causing the PAD to increase more than the PCWP as well as an increase in PVR. Cardiac tamponade would cause elevation and equalization of the CVP, PAD, and PCWP. Left ventricular failure would cause an increase in PAD and PCWP. An MI would not cause any of the above changes, but if there was left ventricular failure or cardiogenic shock that went along with it, there could be increases in the PAD and PCWP.

33) **Correct answer: D** When identifying hemodynamic parameters for the purpose of diagnosis, always remember that an elevated CVP either means fluid overload or an obstruction in the right ventricle. The PAP is a direct indication of left ventricular end-

diastolic pressure. An elevation of the PAP tells you that diastolic clearing is insufficient. The PCWP is indicative of left atrial pressures or left sided preload. Having this number elevated coincides with an elevated PAP. Looking at the hemodynamic parameters and identifying the CI below 2 should immediately suspect a diagnosis of cardiogenic shock. Treatment would be optimizing left ventricular clearing and inotrope.

34) **Correct answer: B** PA pressures are measured through the distal port. It measures PA systolic pressure (PAS) with normal being 20-30mmHg. It also measures PA diastolic pressure (PAD) with normal being 10-15mmHg. This indirectly reflects LV end-diastole pressure.

35) **Correct answer: A** Catheter whip will almost always resemble a large complex V-tach. Catheter whip (or fling) results from movement of the catheter within the vasculature that produces hydrostatic pressure changes at the tip of the catheter that are independent of any changes in hydrostatic pressure within the vessel itself.

36) **Correct answer: C** Central venous pressure (CVP) monitors right atrial pressure and is a direct indication of preload. CVP will always dictate fluid needs. Normal CVP is 2-6mmHg.

37) **Correct answer: D** Elevated PA pressures are a direct indication of afterload (left atrial and ventricular end-diastolic pressures). Mitral valve regurgitation, stenosis, and left ventricular failure are all primary aspects of afterload and left ventricular function.

38) **Correct answer: B** The values of CVP 13, CI 1.4, and PCWP 18, all are an indication of left sided failure. The CVP is high showing that there are high pressures upstream (left side are elevated). The CI is a direct reflection of CO, which tells you the left ventricular function is poor. PCWP is a direct reflection of left ventricular end diastolic pressure

and is elevated. Your diagnosis should be left sided heart failure.
39) **Correct answer: D** Your waveform is showing a right ventricular waveform. You never want your catheter lying in the right ventricle; this could cause V-tach. The proper treatment would be to pull back the catheter into the right atrium/CVP position. Make sure to always deflate the balloon so as to not damage the tricuspid valve. This is a tuff question as it relates to practice in the field, whether you advance it into the pulmonary artery or pull it back into the CVP position will depend on your protocol, knowledge and experience with advancing the catheter.
40) **Correct answer: D** Identifying the dicrotic notch on the left side of the waveform should make you identify that the catheter is located in the RV.
41) **Correct answer: C** Looking at the following hemodynamic parameters can be overwhelming. First, the CVP is a direct indication of preload, with a normal CVP of 2-6mmHg. A CVP of 28 should immediately make you think of an overload state. The CI is showing low and a reflection of cardiac output despite an SVR that is high at 1700. Your PA systolic and diastolic pressures are both high as well as the PCWP. Diagnosis should be cardiogenic shock/left sided failure.
42) **Correct answer: B** Any accumulation of blood around the pericardial sack that is not normal and is of an acute traumatic source will greatly hinder cardiac output. This will put pressure on the atria and ventricles, thus increasing the CVP pressure as well as everything down stream. Therefore, the PAP and PCWP will be greatly elevated. You will see the CVP, PAP and PCWP in this presentation all having a pressure range of 5mmHg from each other because of the equal pressure being placed around the heart. Preload, as well as afterload, will be greatly decreased. Immediate recognition is

essential and a pericardiocentesis is mandatory to relieve the pressure. Surgical repair will then need to take place.

43) **Correct answer: B** Anytime you identify that your patient's PA diastolic pressure is higher than their PCWP, it's an indication of pulmonary hypertension. Pulmonary hypertension is a disease process secondary to an acute hypoxic state, COPD, ARDS, or pulmonary embolus.

Chapter 10 | IABP Therapy

1) **Correct answer: Early Inflation** This timing error is very dangerous. You should have identified that there is no V on the inflation side. The V should have come down to the level of the dicrotic notch. You should have also looked at the deflation side and noticed that there is a V as well. You should always see the U shape. So this patient is in trouble and this timing error will need to be fixed!
2) **Correct answer: Late Inflation & Early Deflation** This timing error is not dangerous. You should have noticed that the dicrotic notch is exposed. This should tell you late inflation!
3) **Correct answer: Early Deflation** This timing error is not dangerous. You should have noticed that the inflation side looks good with the V. The deflation side shows the gradual return to baseline, thus indicating early deflation!
4) **Correct answer: Late Deflation** This timing error is the most dangerous. You should have noticed that the inflation side looks good with the V. The deflation side also has a V. Remember V + V = Late Deflation!
5) **Correct answer: C** Initial set up triggers will always utilize the ECG as the primary trigger. Using the ECG's R wave gives more precise timing in comparison to the dicrotic notch on the A-line. An A-line trigger will be used if the patient has A-fib or there is interference with the ECG. However, A-line use for triggering has limitations and does not time as well.

6) **Correct answer: C** Late deflation is the most harmful timing error because, as the heart starts the systolic phase, the balloon inflation causes excessive stretch and impedes left ventricular ejection and increases afterload. Remember, we are trying to improve diastole filling and coronary artery perfusion during diastole and reducing afterload during systole.
7) **Correct answer: D** If this event happens, it is essential to manually inflate the balloon every 30 minutes to minimize possible clot formation. If this isn't done, when the balloon is removed, you will load the arterial system with emboli and cause further harm or death to your patient.
8) **Correct answer: B** The balloon location should be positioned so that the tip is approximately 1 to 2 cm below the origin of the left subclavian artery and above the renal arteries. If the balloon migrates up and blocks the subclavian artery, you will lose left radial pulses. If it migrates down you will lose renal perfusion and urine output will slow and stop. It is very critical to monitor and check these often.
9) **Correct answer: B** Late deflation is the most ominous timing error because it causes increased pressures that translate to increased after-load and a reduction in coronary artery perfusion.
10) **Correct answer: D** If you ever see rust color flakes in your A-line, this should tell you there has been a balloon rupture. Once blood enters the dry, cold helium rich environment of the IABP balloon, it quickly dries, flakes and changes to a rust or brown color.

11) **Correct answer: A** Your most accurate trigger for IABP operation is going to be your ECG and is timed off the "R" wave. Your secondary form of timing is the A-Line.
12) **Correct answer: B** Migration of the IABP will cause a loss of flow to the renal arteries, decreased renal perfusion, loss of flow to the subclavian arteries and cause loss of circulation to the left arm via the radial artery.
13) **Correct answer: C** Aortic insufficiency, aortic valve failure or stenosis is a contraindication to IABP therapy. Not having an adequate aortic valve will cause insufficient diastolic augmentation during aortic valve closure.
14) **Correct answer: C** The tip should be positioned so that it's approximately 1 to 2 cm below the origin of the left subclavian artery and above the renal arteries. If it migrates up, you will have left subclavian occlusion and lose left radial pulses. If the balloon migrates down, it will impede renal blood flow and urine output will slow and stop. Confirm with x-ray!
15) **Correct answer: D** Early inflation is the second worst timing error. You should identify it by looking at the inflation side of the waveform and seeing the small V. Second, you should have identified late deflation. This is the most ominous timing error that causes increased after-load and decreased coronary artery perfusion. If the balloon is still inflated during the start of the systolic phase it will cause the heart to pump against that increased pressure, thus causing the heart to work harder.
16) **Correct answer: B** Although optimal timing is 1:1, a 1:2 timing is the standard starting timing. It is also best for A-fib, tachycardia and weaning.

17) **Correct answer: D** Intra-aortic balloon pump therapy is used to augment left ventricular diastolic pressures. Augmentation of left ventricular diastolic pressures increase perfusion to the coronary arteries without increasing after-load or the work load of the heart.
18) **Correct answer: A** Helium is used to fill the balloon because it has low density and viscosity allowing the gas to travel through the balloon quickly and reducing the cycling time needed to inflate and deflate the balloon. In addition, if the balloon were to rupture, the helium would be easily dissolved in the body. Helium is also used in refractory hypoxic patients that have narrowing of upper and lower airways. The helium is used as a Heliox 80:20 mixture with oxygen to transport the oxygen molecule down into the swollen airways. The helium can penetrate those lower airways much easier than oxygen alone.
19) **Correct answer: A** This timing location for the diastolic augmentation should always coincide with the closure of the aortic valve. Closure of the aortic valve is identified and timed via the "R" wave that matches the dicrotic notch on the A-line. For timing, the IABP's primary timing method is via the "R" wave in the QRS complex, with the secondary timing method being the A-line.

Chapter 11 | Endocrine Emergencies, Renal & Sepsis

1) **Correct answer: C** This patient is demonstrating a positive Murphy's sign. The pain is elicited when the gallbladder is trapped between the hand and the liver upon palpation. In order to be truly positive, the same maneuver should not elicit pain when performed on the (L) side.
2) **Correct answer: B** This patient's complaints are consistent with a positive Kehr's sign, which indicates the presence of blood in the peritoneal cavity. This is a classic symptom with a splenic rupture and the spleen is the most common abdominal organ injured in blunt trauma.
3) **Correct answer: D** With patients in DKA, it is essential to allow the patient to continue to compensate. Remember the rule, for every 10mmHg increase in PaCO2, you will have a decrease in pH by 0.08. If we were to paralyze them and take away their compensatory mechanism, their PaCO2 would significantly increase thus dropping the pH to levels of nonviable life. Proper ventilator strategies in this situation would be to place them on SIMV and give moderate sedation to allow the patient the ability to continue their compensatory drive. Option C would not be as beneficial due to AC and higher Vt.
4) **Correct answer: B** An aldosterone substitute would only encourage further water reabsorption. Vasopressin acts as an antidiuretic and will increase water permeability in the renal tubular cells thus decreasing urine volume further. These patients do not need more fluid, they need diuresis and fluid restriction.

5) **Correct answer: A** There is failure "before" the kidneys due to the hypovolemia. The kidneys are not being perfused enough therefore is not diuresing.
6) **Correct answer: C** A decrease in DTRs indicates a drop in the pH and worsening metabolic acidosis leading to DKA. A urine pH less than 6 indicates that the kidneys are excreting acid. An increase in the bicarb indicates improvement in current acidotic state and potassium levels are expected to decrease as acidosis is corrected and potassium is shifted back into the intracellular space.
7) **Correct answer: C** Remember DI is caused by adequate or no ADH production or release from the pituitary gland. This can be caused from a head injury or the use of phenytoin (Dilantin). The other choices are for DKA.
8) **Correct answer: C** Appendicitis is lower abdominal pain, so that can be ruled out. GI perforation and hemorrhage do not go along with the respiratory and diaphragm changes and hepatitis is included in that as well. Remember, Cullen's sign, alcoholism, and upper abdominal pain equals pancreatitis, which can lead to sepsis and ARDS.
9) **Correct answer: B** 0.9% NS is the best initial fluid for resuscitation of dehydration and hyperglycemia. LR is incorrect because the presence of lactate is not desirable in someone with profound acidosis. 0.45% NS is hypotonic and will provide less BP support and will not correct dehydration. 3% NS creates an osmotic shift from intracellular water into the intravascular space, making dehydration worse.

10) **Correct answer: B** SIADH is the overproduction or release of ADH which results in increased serum retention with secondary water retention due to the stimulation of aldosterone receptors in the nephrons. This results in a dilutional hyponatremic state.
11) **Correct answer: C** This patient meets the criteria for severe sepsis with evidence of organ dysfunction and hypotension. The patient has not received any treatments at this point, so septic shock cannot be defined.
12) **Correct answer: Rationale** CVP 8-12mmHg; MAP >65 mmHg; UO >0.5 mL/kg/hr; SvO2 of 65-70%; Blood cultures; IV antibiotic administration ASAP (preferably within the 1st hour)
13) **Correct answer: C** Serum osmolality is a measure to check the balance between water and the chemicals dissolved in it. It is an indicator showing dehydration or overhydration. Normal is 275-295 mOsm/kg. Elevated levels occur in the presence of dehydration. All other instances would occur with a decreased serum osmolality level.
14) **Correct answer: D** According to the Society of Critical Care Medicine Consensus Panel, fluid resuscitation should be at 30 mL/kg with a recommendation of crystalloids being used.
15) **Correct answer: D** Diabetes insipidus occurs from a low level of ADH, so the patient loses large amounts of water. This causes an increase in serum Na+, an increase in serum osmolality and an increase in urinary output with a decrease in urinary osmolality resulting from a decrease in urinary concentration.
16) **Correct answer: A** These patients are dehydrated and really need the fluids. Part of the management with both of these conditions is replenishing the fluids along with managing the hyperglycemia.

17) **Correct answer: C** Respiratory failure is common, usually in the first 72 hours, followed by hepatic failure and then renal failure.
18) **Correct answer: B** Hyperglycemia is due to the insulin deficiency found in type I diabetics. The elevated blood sugar levels leads to a hypertonic diuresis, state of dehydration, and elevation in the serum osmolality. There is an increase in the breakdown of fats and proteins for energy, which leads to an increase in ketones in the blood, leading to a state of ketoacidosis. The acidotic environment causes a shift of potassium to move out of the cell and into the serum causing hyperkalemia.
19) **Correct answer: C** Due to the patient's cracked lips, hypotension, and tachycardia, you would assume he is in a state of dehydration (hypovolemia). Administration of fluids will prevent further problems and hypovolemic shock. Also, replacement of any lost electrolytes will help prevent further problems or deterioration.
20) **Correct answer: B** With DI, the classic symptoms are increased urination with a low specific gravity. The patient has normal serum glucose, so diabetes development would not be appropriate. With SIADH, the patient's urinary output would be decreased and the specific gravity would be increased.
21) **Correct answer: C** DI occurs after there is a decrease in the amount of ADH that is being secreted. This leads to a state of polyuria because the body has no ADH to tell it to reabsorb water and sodium. With polyuria, the body gets rid of water but not as much sodium so it results in a state of dilutional hypernatremia. Also, the serum osmolality is increased because there are more electrolytes in the serum than water to balance that. The specific

gravity of the urine decreased because the urine contains more free water than electrolytes.

22) **Correct answer: B** Electrical burns will cause destruction of the muscles causing myoglobin to appear in the urine. This can cause acute tubular necrosis and further renal failure if not treated appropriately. The goal of treatment is to flush the myoglobin out with the use of fluids, usually NS, and a diuretic, which is usually mannitol. The urine should be kept alkaline, with the use of bicarbonate, to increase excretion of the myoglobin.

23) **Correct answer: D** For a patient with no pre-existing diseases such as HTN, the CVP target would be 8-12mmHg, but with patients with long-standing HTN or left ventricular hypertrophy, this measurement is going to be slightly higher at 12-15mmHg.

24) **Correct answer: C** According to the Society of Critical Care Medicine Consensus Panel, the endpoint for mixed venous oxygen saturation should be 65-70%. This is going to be the quickest way to identify trends in treatment in a positive or negative way. This is a marker of true tissue oxygenation being a venous measurement.

25) **Correct answer: D** The most common cause of ATN in a patient that's experienced a crush injury is myoglobinuria. Rhabdomyolysis is an acute process secondary to massive myoglobin release. Myoglobin is the oxygen transport molecule for muscles. It is not intended to be released from the muscles and if this occurs, it is toxic to the kidneys causing acute renal failure and inducing intratubular cast formation. The normal treatment for this patient would be volume resuscitation with the goal of urinary output of 100 mL/hr. Also, the administration of sodium bicarbonate infusion along with some form of a diuretic, either Lasix or Mannitol to induce diuresis would be done.

26) **Correct answer: B** Although MODS can occur with sepsis, it does not have to. It can occur without the presence of an infectious process. The definition of MODS does not require complete cessation of function of organs, but there has to be two or more organs involved to be classified as MODS.
27) **Correct answer: C** Due to the initiation of vasopressin and the effects of systemic vasoconstriction that occurs with this medication, myocardial ischemia has most likely occurred. When giving vasopressin in this type of patient presentation, nitroglycerin is concurrently administered to prevent the adverse side effect of vasoconstriction.
28) **Correct answer: C** In the hyperdynamic stage of sepsis, contractility and CO are initially increased in an attempt to compensate. As sepsis progresses to septic shock, preload and afterload decrease due to the massive vasodilation that takes place in this disease process. When looking at hemodynamic parameters in septic shock, you will see all parameters (CVP, PAD, PCWP, and CI) decreased.
29) **Correct answer: A** Infection is the most common cause of DKA in insulin dependent patients due to the increased need for insulin during these periods. Remember, in patient's with an increased oxygen demand, the liver is secreting enormous amounts of glycogen for the process of ATP production. Due to the insufficiency of insulin already in this patient, they require more insulin than normal to keep up with the production of increased glucose.
30) **Correct answer: B** In the spectrum of endocrine emergencies, thyroid storm ranks as one of the most critical illnesses. Recognition and appropriate management of life-threatening thyrotoxicosis is vital

to prevent the high morbidity and mortality that accompanies this disorder.
31) **Correct answer: B** pH and K+ have an inverse relationship. For every 0.10 increase in the pH, you anticipate the K+ to decrease by 0.6. They will always move opposite of each other.
32) **Correct answer: D** In DKA patients, you expect to see a state of metabolic acidosis. The patient's pH is normally <7.3 and a decreased CO2 due to the patient attempting to compensate by blowing off excess CO2 (Kussmaul respirations).
33) **Correct answer: B** Cullen's sign consists of superficial edema and bruising around the umbilicus. It can occur with acute pancreatitis, bleeding from blunt trauma, bleeding from a ruptured abdominal aortic aneurysm, or bleeding from a ruptured ectopic pregnancy.
34) **Correct answer: C** Sandostatin (Octreotide) reduces secretion of fluids by the intestines and pancreas as well as reduces GI motility and inhibits contraction of the gallbladder. It causes vasoconstriction in the blood vessels and reduces portal vessel pressures in bleeding varices.
35) **Correct answer: C** In a patient suffering from DKA, there is an absolute insulin deficiency that causes glycogenolysis and gluconeogenesis. The gluconeogenesis causes the incomplete breakdown of free fatty acids, which result in ketones in the blood and urine. In HHNK, there is a relative insulin deficiency that causes glycogenolysis but does not cause gluconeogenesis. Therefore, test for ketones are positive in the DKA patient and negative in the HHNK patient respectively.

Chapter 12 | Trauma Management

1) **Correct answer: C** This is a classic FP-C / CFRN question for cardiac tamponade. In real life context, the JVD and narrowing pulse pressure are going to be your ticket to diagnosis. None of us are good at listening to heart tones and in flight that will be difficult.
2) **Correct answer: A** No rationale provided
3) **Correct answer: B** Kehr's sign is indicative of splenic injury or rupture that has referred pain to the left shoulder. Match this to MOI and use it for differential diagnosis for medical presentations that present with abdominal pain with the risk or diagnosis of mononucleosis.
4) **Correct answer: A** The consensus formula is the new standard in burn fluid resuscitation management. You should still know the Parkland formula. However, just know that the consensus formula is the Parkland formula cut in half.
5) **Correct answer: C** Urine output is essential in any patient. A patient that is producing urine is a patient that is perfusing. Urine output should be aimed at 30-50mL/hr. In patients with a risk of rhabdomyolysis, urine output should be aimed at 100mL/hr.
6) **Correct answer: A** Rule of 9's state that the head accounts for 9% with the face and head combined, each arm is 9% totaling 18% with each arm burned. Total BSA is 27%.
7) **Correct answer: C** The modified formula states: **Kg x TBSA x 2-4 mL = volume/24 hours**. Administer half of the total fluids during first eight hours post burn. Administer a quarter of total fluids during

second eight hours post burn. Then administer a quarter of the total fluids during the third eight hours post burn.
8) **Correct answer: A** All of the above answers are correct except for vasopressin. All correct answers are used to increase urine output and to flush the kidneys. Vasopressin would do just the opposite and cause water retention.
9) **Correct answer: B** The Parkland formula states: **Kg x TBSA x 4mL = volume/24 hours. 90kg X 65 X 4 = 23,400[23,400/2 = 11,700 in the first 8 hours].** Administer half of the total fluids during the first eight hours post burn. Next administer a quarter of the total fluids during the second eight hours post burn. Then administer a quarter of the total fluids during the third eight hours post burn.
10) **Correct answer: C** The Parkland formula states: **Kg x TBSA x 4mL = volume/24 hours. 70kg X 45 X 4 = 12,600mL [12,600/2 = 6,300 in the first eight hours].** The question asked how much the patient should get in the first 24 hours. **= 12,600 mL**
11) **Correct answer: B** With any burn patient, remember you can have significant K+ shifts. Always watch this and with any transfer with burns >12 hours, be ready to treat any hyperkalemia that results in ECG changes.
12) **Correct answer: A** The Parkland formula states: **Kg x TBSA x 4mL = volume/24 hours. 72kg X 31.5 X 4 = 9,072 [9,072/2 = 4,536 in the first eight hours].** Administer half of the total fluids during the first eight hours post burn. Next, administer a quarter of the total fluids during the second eight hours post burn. Finally, administer a quarter of the total fluids during the third eight hours post burn.

13) **Correct answer: C** Acceleration-deceleration injuries cause a shearing tear of the aortic arch. Approximately 80% of patients that die within minutes of the accident have this type of large vessel tear.
14) **Correct answer: C** Commotio cordis is caused by unexpected blunt force trauma that is non-penetrating to the left lateral chest or pericardium during the vulnerable state of ventricular repolarization causing a fatal ventricular dysrhythmia and sudden cardiac death.
15) **Correct answer: C** A positive Kehr's sign is left shoulder pain which is indicative of a ruptured spleen. Along with the patient's positive Cullen's sign, which is ecchymosis around the umbilicus that is indicative of intraperitoneal bleeding secondary to liver and spleen lacerations, the patient presentation would indicate splenic injury or rupture.
16) **Correct answer: B** Recommended urinary output for the adult patient should be 30-50 mL/hr or 0.5-1 mL/kg/hr. This is an important indicator of volume status. If a patient is suffering from crush or burn injuries and has secondary rhabdomyolysis, urine output should be maintained at a minimum of 100mL/hr.
17) **Correct answer: D** Rhabdomyolysis occurs when damaged skeletal muscle tissue breaks down causing damage to the kidneys. Hyperthermia and prolonged seizure activity can both lead to this development. The elevated CK is the first indicator along with increases in the BUN and Cr indicating kidney damage.
18) **Correct answer: D** Bicarbonate administration may help alleviate acidosis and make the urine more alkaline preventing cast formation in the kidneys. When alkalizing the urine, the pH should be kept at 6.5 or above.

19) **Correct answer: D** The earliest lab value that identifies muscle damage and release of myoglobin is going to be CK. Creatine kinase is an enzyme that is present in all the muscles of the body and is a catalyst in the energy conversion process. Creatine kinase is used in the body in two types - for the muscles and for the brain.
20) **Correct answer: C** The infusion of unwarmed or inadequately warmed intravenous (IV) fluids and cold blood may contribute to the multiple adverse consequences associated with hypothermia including: cardiac arrhythmia, hemostasis abnormalities from impaired platelet function and impaired coagulation cascade, peripheral vasoconstriction, dehydration, decreased oxygen delivery to tissues, which impairs oxidative killing of bacteria by neutrophils, and reduction in the deposition of collagen during wound healing, increased red cell release of potassium plus metabolic acidosis, and citrate toxicity (with blood component transfusion).
21) **Correct answer: B** If your patient has a bronchial tree tear, often times it's at the carina. If you note on your assessment that you have subcutaneous air and decreasing SaO2, the proper treatment is to advance the ETT past the carina for a right main stem intubation. This will secure an airway past the bronchial tear and allow you to ventilate the right lung. Even though this causes a right to left shunt, it's better than nothing and may buy you time.
22) **Correct answer: B** Myoglobinuria, if left untreated, will result in acute tubular necrosis and profound renal failure. The only time myoglobin is found in the bloodstream is when it is released following muscle injury. It is an abnormal finding, and can be diagnostically relevant when found in the blood. Myoglobinuria is the presence of myoglobin in the urine, usually associated

with rhabdomyolysis or muscle destruction, and is lethal if left untreated.

23) **Correct answer: A** 1mg/dL increase in the hemoglobin and 3% increase in the hematocrit is the standard ratio of increase with administration of one unit of packed red cells. Another good way to identify your H&H ratio is to multiply your Hgb x 3, which should equal your Hct.

24) **Correct answer: D** Platelets, cryoprecipitate, and FFP are the first line treatment to slow the DIC process. When patients are given massive transfusions of NS and PRBCs, all of their clotting factors get washed out. On top of that, the body's response to injury is to start an inflammatory cascade in the attempt to heal. This massive inflammatory cascade leads to the formation of small blood clots inside the blood vessels throughout the body. As the small clots consume coagulation proteins and platelets, normal coagulation is disrupted and abnormal bleeding occurs from the skin, the gastrointestinal tract, the respiratory tract and surgical wounds. The small clots also disrupt normal blood flow to organs (such as the kidneys), which may malfunction as a result. Regardless of the triggering event of DIC, once initiated, the pathophysiology of DIC is similar in all conditions. There have been two current studies that have proven beneficial for these trauma patients where massive hemorrhage and transfusion occurs. Administration of tranexamic acid (TXA), within the first hour of the traumatic event with potential hemorrhage, has resulted in a lower incidence of DIC and reduced mortality.

25) **Correct answer: C** The classical findings on a chest x-ray will be widened mediastinum, apical cap, and displacement of the trachea. A normal chest x-ray does not exclude transection, but will diagnose conditions such as pneumothorax or hemothorax.

26) **Correct answer: B** Often, diagnosis in the field of a hemothorax is difficult. This should be treated as a pneumothorax until proven otherwise. A massive hemothorax can accumulate up to 1500cc of blood in the chest cavity. Maintaining a good MAP of 65mmHg to allow for tissue perfusion and good oxygenation is your primary goal. If a chest tube is placed, only clamp the chest tube if you have an initial blood loss of 1500cc of blood, otherwise never clamp the chest tube.
27) **Correct answer: D** Citrate is the anticoagulant used in blood products and is rapidly metabolized by the liver in normal situations. Rapid administration of large quantities of stored blood may cause hypocalcaemia and hypomagnesaemia when citrate binds with calcium and magnesium. This can result in myocardial depression or coagulopathy. Patients most at risk are those with liver dysfunction or neonates with immature liver function having rapid large volume transfusions. Slowing or temporarily stopping the transfusion allows citrate to be metabolized. Replacement therapy may be required for symptomatic hypocalcaemia or hypomagnesaemia. Calcium gluconate or chloride is going to be your first line treatment after stopping the transfusion. This will increase inotrope and improve vasotone by bringing the hypocalcaemia to a normal level.
28) **Correct answer: B** Fracture of the 1st-3rd ribs should indicate a great amount of force. Aortic disruption along with C1-C2 fracture and scapular fractures can be associated with this amount of force and mechanism.
29) **Correct answer: D** Correct placement for chest tube insertion is the 4th ICS anterior axillary. This is an important landmark. Migration down lower into the 5th or 6th ICS can cause liver or spleen injuries and misplacement.

30) **Correct answer: C** Anytime you see a trauma patient that has no compensatory mechanisms manifesting, think neurogenic shock. With the age of the patient, along with the hypotension and bradycardia, this is classic neurogenic shock. This is classified as a vasogenic shock and if you had available hemodynamic readings you would see a low CVP, low PA pressure, low PCWP, low SVR and a normal to high CO.
31) **Correct answer: D** Beck's triad is indicative of muffled heart tones, narrowing pulse pressures and JVD. In an increased ICP patient, you would see Cushing's triad in the patient that is herniating.
32) **Correct answer: B** Thrombophlebitis is an inflammation of a vein, usually in your legs, that becomes swollen due to a blood clot. A blood clot is a solid formation of blood cells that stick together. Thrombophlebitis can occur in veins near the surface of your skin or deeper down in one of your muscles.
33) **Correct answer: A** When we look at mechanism and potential injury patterns associated with different types of collisions, rear impact collisions will most likely be associated with c-spine injuries from the axial loading forces.
34) **Correct answer: C** Great vessel laceration is a common cause of death in trauma patients. Aortic disruption is the most common cause due to the shearing injury that occurs from the deceleration forces seen in high force accidents.
35) **Correct answer: D** Tension pneumothorax will cause tracheal deviation to the unaffected side and breath sounds will be decreased to absent on the affected side. Although tracheal deviation is a very late sign and something that is not easily identifiable, for testing purposes this is a common question and answer.

36) **Correct answer: C** While all of these could be the cause of myocardial contusion, the most likely cause is from an MVC. Blunt chest trauma in the MVC setting is common, and can occur as a result of hitting the steering wheel or the up and over forces in a motorcycle accident.
37) **Correct answer: B** This is a positive Kehr's sign and can occur with a ruptured spleen. This sign is suspicious especially after a traumatic event involving rib fractures on the (L) side.
38) **Correct answer: C** Beck's triad includes hypotension, jugular neck distension, and muffled heart sounds. In cardiac tamponade, other clinical findings could include: pulsus paradoxus and equalizations of cardiac pressures, where the CVP, PAP, and PCWP are increased and within 5 mmHg of each other.
39) **Correct answer: C** When identifying potential types of shock in your trauma patients, always think about hemorrhage and potential secondary problems associated with losing large amounts of blood. Hgb concentrations are essential for oxygen carrying capacity and should be watched closely. The patient will become tissue hypoxic quickly and anaerobic metabolism will ensue.
40) **Correct answer: B** FiO2 will improve oxygenation in all situations. However, when used in conjunction with PEEP, it will provide optimal results. Remember, oxygen is a true biological toxin and the body doesn't need high amounts. We live just fine on 21%. Normal cellular metabolism involves the addition of 4 single electrons to the O2 molecule. During normal partial pressure (100 mmHg), 95% of the molecules will be reduced to H20 and 5% will be partially reduced (toxic metabolites or free radicals [FR]). FRs leak into the cytosol, and out from the cell. FRs cause much of the cellular damage seen in O2 toxicity. The first symptom will usually be

substernal chest pain that is exacerbated by deep breathing. A dry cough and dyspnea will follow.

41) **Correct answer: D** If you look at this patients hemodynamic numbers, it should steer you in the direction that the cardiac output is through the roof, but the SVR is really low. This inhibits the delivery of oxygen to the tissues. Essentially, the perfusion gradient is significantly hindered, so less oxygen is delivered. We can identify this by using the Fick Formula *(VO2 =[1.34 x Hgb x (SvO2)] +0.003 x PO2 = CvO2)*. This patient is also febrile and has the beginning look of sepsis. In sepsis, the body has an inability to extract the oxygen that is delivered. This results in blood returning to the right side of the heart with more oxygen still attached to the hemoglobin.

Chapter 13 | Neurological Injuries

1) **Correct answer: C** To calculate the CPP you need to figure the MAP. MAP= ([2DBP] + SBP) / 3. CPP = MAP - ICP. This patient has a MAP of 110mmHg – ICP 23 = CPP 87.
2) **Correct answer: D** Brown-Sequard syndrome is a rare injury that affects the hemisection of the cord (usually cervical region), and causes ipsilateral loss of motor position and vibratory sense with contralateral loss of pain and temperature perception.
3) **Correct answer: A** This is a classic advanced certification exam question. Remember, epidural bleeds will have a period of initial consciousness followed by a period of lucidity and then go unresponsive. Often, that last phase of unresponsiveness will lead to airway difficulties, clenched teeth, and increased ICP.
4) **Correct answer: B** Cushing's triad is an ominous sign and not often seen in the early management of our patients. This is a clear indication of severe ICP and if left untreated leads to herniation and death.
5) **Correct answer: A** Diffuse axonal injury (DAI) is an ominous diagnosis and is difficult to identify. CT and MRI scans will show unidentifiable damage. DAI is an injury that causes severe shearing of the axons of the nerve cells throughout the brain.
6) **Correct answer: A** You first need to determine the MAP pressure. Standard ICP = 0-15mmHg. MAP = ([2(Diastolic)] + Systolic)/3. CCP = MAP – ICP. In this problem your MAP = 73. CCP = 73 - 28 = 45mmHg.

7) **Correct answer: A** With any patient suffering from stroke like symptoms with a secondary seizure, you should always suspect intracerebral hemorrhage. This condition would be an absolute contraindication for fibrinolytic therapy.
8) **Correct answer: C** CPP should be at least 70 mmHg to ensure adequate blood flow to the brain. (CPP = MAP - ICP). Remember that 25% of your CO goes directly to oxygenate your brain. Maintaining the proper CPP is essential for proper oxygen delivery to the nervous system.
9) **Correct answer: B** A stellate skull fracture occurs with multiple linear fractures radiating from the site of impact.
10) **Correct answer: C** CPP = MAP – ICP
11) **Correct answer: B** Diffuse axonal injury (DAI) is a type of traumatic brain injury where damage occurs in a widespread area rather than a focal area. DAI is difficult to detect because the CT will not show any major changes.
12) **Correct answer: B** Epidural hematomas occur when blood accumulates between the dura mater and the skull. Epidural bleeding is rapid because it is usually from an artery. The hallmark symptom is the patient may regain consciousness and appear completely normal only to descend suddenly and rapidly into an unconscious state.
13) **Correct answer: D** Basilar skull fractures may present with CSF rhinorrhea, otorrhea, Battle sign and "raccoon eyes". Facial palsy, nystagmus and facial numbness are secondary and can occur due to the involvement of cranial nerves V, VI, and VII respectively.
14) **Correct answer: C** The transducer should be leveled at the point of the patient's face which corresponds to the Foramen of Monro. This is the outer canthus of the eye. As with any other invasive transducers, the major point to remember is that it

must always be leveled, so pick your mark and stick with it!

15) **Correct answer: B** Brown-Sequard syndrome results in a loss of sensation and motor function caused by a lateral hemisection of the spinal cord. This is associated with: ipsilateral paralysis below the level of the lesion, positive Babinski sign ipsilateral to the lesion, ipsilateral loss of tactile discrimination, vibratory, and position sensation below the level of the lesion, and contralateral loss of pain and temperature sensation.

16) **Correct answer: B** In this presentation, using a medication that will work on reducing afterload and systemic vascular resistance is essential. Bringing the diastolic pressure below 100-120 is the goal. Be careful to ensure you know the patient's normal ranges and only bring down the pressure to a point that stops the symptoms.

17) **Correct answer: C** In the presence of a Sub-Arachnoid Hemorrhage, it essential to maintain systolic BP at 140 systolic. Unlike the treatment goals associated with an intracerebral hemorrhage, systolic BP needs to be 160 mmHg due to the location of the bleed and the required MAP needed to perfuse that level of the brain. In contrast, Sub Arachnoid Hemorrhages have a very high probability for re-bleeding. As such, the systolic BP and associated MAP need to be lower.

Chapter 14 – Toxicology

1) **Correct answer: A** TCAs inhibit the reabsorption of dopamine, epinephrine, and norepinephrine. They work in a manner similar to cocaine. Therefore, erratic behavior seen in cocaine overdose, are frequently seen with TCA OD as well.
2) **Correct answer: C** Although current ACLS guidelines still recommend Atropine for early treatment, resolution of symptoms are not expected. It is still recommended to attempt to eliminate any other factors such as increased vagal tone.
3) **Correct answer: B** TCA OD will present with tachycardia progressing to QRS widening with worsening toxicity. This will eventually lead to VT, VF, or Torsades de Pointes.
4) **Correct answer: D** The metabolites of acetaminophen usually take 24-48 hours to accumulate within the liver. This is when RUQ pain becomes the predominant symptom that presents.
5) **Correct answer: B** Hyperkalemia is the usual electrolyte abnormality precipitated by digoxin toxicity. Hyperkalemia may be associated with acute renal failure that subsequently precipitates digoxin toxicity.
6) **Correct answer: Rationale** First: Calcium Chloride (500-1000mg) IV over 5-10mins. Insulin and glucose. Sodium bicarbonate, Albuterol, and Lasix. Kayexalate and magnesium sulfate as needed as well.
7) **Correct answer: D** Cyanide binds to cytochrome c oxidase in the electron transfer chain, thus inhibiting oxygen conversion to water and stopping ATP synthesis. As a result, the chain can no longer

produce ATP, which quickly leads to both CNS and cardiac insults. It takes 1-15 minutes to cause death. This causes us to move from an aerobic state to an anaerobic state. Any patients that have sustained prolonged periods in house fires that are hypoxic, despite oxygenation therapy, should be suspected of having cyanide toxicity.

8) **Correct answer: C** Aspirin is acetylsalicylic acid, which causes a respiratory stimulant effect leading to respiratory alkalosis. It also causes a direct metabolic acidosis due to being an acid as well.
9) **Correct answer: C** The sympathetic nervous system is responsible for the signs and symptoms of hypoglycemia. Medications that block the sympathetic system, such as beta-blockers, could potentially prevent an individual from experiencing these symptoms. Symptoms include: tachycardia, diaphoresis and nervousness. Beta-blockers such as metoprolol can cause patients to become severely hypoglycemic without being able to identify the symptoms early on.
10) **Correct answer: D** Sodium affects phase zero on the action potential which is responsible for depolarization. Calcium, magnesium and potassium all work on phase 2 and 3 of the action potential, which is responsible for repolarization. Low levels of calcium, magnesium and potassium will affect phase 2 and 3 of the action potential by slowing repolarization causing prolonged QT segments.
11) **Correct answer: D** Amitriptyline (Elavil) is a TCA, which causes QT prolongation by inhibiting sodium uptake and may result in Torsades de Pointes or other arrhythmias.
12) **Correct answer: A** Salicylate has a respiratory stimulant effect, which will lead to respiratory alkalosis. It's also an acid and causes metabolic acidosis later in the presentation.

Chapter 15 | OB/GYN Emergencies

1) **Correct answer: C** Effacement refers to the thickness of the cervix, with no effacement meaning that the cervix hasn't thinned, 50% effacement meaning it has thinned halfway, etc.
2) **Correct answer: C** This is a common test question, knowing that Mauriceu's maneuver is the standard for any breech delivery.
3) **Correct answer: D** With any neonate suffering from poor variability, always think about anything that causes hypoxia or prematurity.
4) **Correct answer: A** Sinusoidal patterns are the most ominous sign. This occurs due to anemia and severe fetal distress. During contraction, the HR will not rise concurrently. Oxygen carrying capacity is deficient and hypoxia ensues. C-Section is the first line treatment.
5) **Correct answer: B** Brethine is used for pre-term labor only. The other choices can be used for treatment of PIH with Hydralazine being the first choice.
6) **Correct answer: B** First stage: The time of the onset of true labor until the cervix is 10 cm dilated. Second stage: After the cervix is fully dilated until the baby is delivered. Third stage: Delivery of the placenta.
7) **Correct answer: B** Acute toxicity needs to be treated with CaCl aggressively. If you had a patient with chronic toxicity, you could give a loop diuretic because $MgSO_4$ is easily eliminated via the renal system.

8) **Correct answer: C** Uterine rupture can occur with trauma. In a complete uterine rupture, the fetus may be palpated easily over the abdomen. This is an emergency with a high mortality/morbidity for both the fetus and the mother.
9) **Correct answer: D** The Mauriceau's maneuver is utilized in cases of breech delivery. The procedure includes one person applying supra-pubic pressure on the mother while another person inserts a hand into the vagina, palpating the fetal maxilla using the index and middle finger and gently pressing on the maxilla, bringing the neck to a moderate flexion position to help facilitate birth.
10) **Correct answer: A** A sinusoidal FHR pattern is fixed, uniform fluctuations of the FHR and characterized by absence of variability. Sinusoidal FHR pattern can be associated with the following fetal conditions: chronic fetal anemia, usually from Rh sensitization, acute, intrapartum asphyxia, fetal-maternal hemorrhage, or in-utero, fetal hemorrhage.
11) **Correct answer: D** Magnesium toxicity results in a sharp drop in BP and respiratory paralysis along with the disappearance of DTRs. IV administration of 500-1000mg of 10% calcium chloride usually reverses the effects of magnesium.
12) **Correct answer: C** HELLP syndrome is a life-threatening OB complication from pre-eclampsia. It can occur during the later stages of pregnancy or even after childbirth. It includes hemolysis, elevated liver enzymes, and low platelet count.
13) **Correct answer: D** Pitocin should be the first drug of choice followed by Methergine to try to stop post-partum hemorrhage. PRBCs or FFP may be required for fluid resuscitation but getting the bleeding to stop is of top priority at this moment.

14) **Correct answer: B** A deceleration is a decrease in the FHR below the baseline. A late deceleration will be to the right of the contraction with the lowest point of the deceleration occurring after the peak of the contraction. Late decelerations occur when a fall in the fetal oxygen level causes reflex constriction of blood vessels in an attempt to divert more blood flow to vital organs of the fetus. The constriction of the blood vessels causes HTN that stimulates a vagal response, which slows the HR.
15) **Correct answer: B** PIH is the development of new HTN in a pregnant woman after 20 weeks of gestation, and consists of high blood pressure, edema due to fluid retention, and proteinuria.
16) **Correct answer: D** Shoulder dystocia occurs after the delivery of the head, when the anterior shoulder cannot pass below the pubic symphysis and requires manipulation. This is an OB emergency and fetal demise can occur if the infant is not delivered due to cord compression within the birth canal. McRobert's manuever involves hyperflexing the mother's legs tightly to her abdomen, which causes the pelvis to widen and flattens the lumbar spine.
17) **Correct answer: D** Magnesium sulfate can help delay labor by inhibiting uterine muscle contractions.
18) **Correct answer: B** Variability is affected by incomplete development of the ANS and plays a part between the parasympathetic and sympathetic systems.
19) **Correct answer: A** DIC can occur in abruptio placentae due to abnormal hemorrhage tendencies and the systemic activation of the coagulation cascade system.

FlightBridgeED, LLC
Chapter 16 | Pediatric & Neonates

1) **Correct answer: B** Transposition of the great vessels is a severe diagnosis for any neonate. It's often associated with VSD and/or PDA patency. It's essential for the PDA to remain patent for the survival of the baby. Often times they will surgical cause a VSD just to provide some oxygen rich blood to flow through the body. These patients are hypoxic and very sick.
2) **Correct answer: C** This is a quick calculation for determining tube size on the fly. You can also use the broselow tape or the baby's pinky finger.
3) **Correct answer: B** Prostaglandin can cause significant respiratory depression and apnea in most neonates. Because of this, it's always beneficial to intubate and place these babies on the vent. Remember to always calculate your O2 because too much oxygen will cause PDA closure. With these neonates, survival is dependent on PDA patency until surgical intervention is completed.
Calculation equation:
$$\frac{\%FiO2 \times P1}{P2} = FiO2 \text{ @ new altitude}$$
   - P1 = Current barometric pressure
   - P2 = New barometric pressure at altitude
4) **Correct answer: C** Neonates and pediatrics compensate well. Remember that you will only see decompensation after 25% blood loss. In a neonate that may only 10-20mLs.
5) **Correct answer: C** Waddell's triad is an injury pattern associated with the child turning toward the car prior to impact. This causes head, chest, abdominal and lower extremity injuries that are often severe.

6) **Correct answer: D** Subtle seizure activity is the most common presentation with neonates. They do not present with standard grand mal, full body seizures. The mouth, tongue and bicycling motion, eye deviation and blinking are the most common.
7) **Correct answer: A** Subtle seizures consist of repetitive mouth/tongue movements, bicycling, eye deviation and blinking. Clonic seizures include repetitive jerky movements of limbs. Tonic seizures may resemble posturing or tonic extension seen in older patients. Myoclonic seizures include multiple jerking motions, usually of the upper extremities.
8) **Correct answer: C** Pulmonary arterial vasoconstriction keeps blood from flowing through the fetal lungs and causes oxygenation to take place in the placenta. At birth, pulmonary adaptation occurs after a complex series of events switches respiration from the placenta to the lungs.
9) **Correct answer: C** Stress on a neonate can present in many different ways. One of those would be the baby suddenly starts hiccoughing, yawning or sneezing multiple times. Although these things can be found normally in the neonate, with distress these things will occur multiple times in a row and all of a sudden.
10) **Correct answer: A** Subtle seizure activity can present in many forms in the neonate and infant. Increasing HR and BP as well as eye fluttering, mouth movements and bicycling actions are also signs of seizure activity within the neonate. You may also see an increase in irritability and decrease in SaO2 during seizure activity.
11) **Correct answer: B** Surfactant is absent in very premature babies and is required to keep the lungs inflated and keep them from sticking. Surfactant helps keep the alveoli open. Without sufficient

surfactant, alveolar collapse, atelectasis trauma, respiratory distress can ensue.
12) **Correct answer: C** In some cases, a patent PDA is beneficial to the neonate and may prolong their life until surgical correction is possible. Prostaglandin administration allows the ductus arteriosus to remain open. Indomethacin blocks prostaglandin production and is used for closure of PDA.
13) **Correct answer: C** Apnea is a common side effect of prostaglandin therapy. However, PDA patency is essential. Because of this side effect, intubation is a must prior to transport. Other common side effects seen may include: flushing, bradycardia, and/or hypotension.
14) **Correct answer: C** Patients that suffer from tetralogy of fallot have multiple issues. Most often, they suffer from a VSD, stenotic pulmonary valve, RV hypertrophy and a pulmonary artery outflow obstruction. PDA patency is essential. Administration of oxygen needs to be minimal along with PGE-1 administration throughout transport. Often the biggest side affect to PGE-1 administration is apnea. As such, intubation is essential prior to transport. Long-term treatment is dilation of the pulmonary artery to alleviate the PA outflow obstruction and surgical repair of the VSD.
15) **Correct answer: C** Tetralogy of fallot is a right-to-left shunt allowing blood to flow from the right heart to the left heart. Tetralogy of fallot results in four defects including: pulmonary stenosis, overriding aorta, right ventricular hypertrophy, and ventricular septal defect.
16) **Correct answer: B** Prior to birth, the placenta is a major source of prostaglandin to keep the PDA open. At birth, pulmonary vascular resistance decreases and blood flows directly from the right ventricle into the lungs. Normal respiration and oxygen tension increases as well causing closure of the PDA.

17) **Correct answer: D** Choanal atresia is a narrowing or blockage of tissue in the nasal airways. These patients will have difficulty breathing and inability to nurse and breath at the same time. Diagnosis is made by attempting to pass a small suction catheter through the nares. Surgical intervention is indicated to repair and remove the blockage in the back of the nasal passages.
18) **Correct answer: D** VSD is one of the most common congenital heart defects, and occurs when there is a hole in the septum between the left and right ventricles.
19) **Correct answer: C** Proper ETT sizing for pediatric patients should be calculated using: (Age + 16) / 4
20) **Correct answer: C** Depth of insertion of an ETT should be approximately 3x that of the ETT size.
21) **Correct answer: B** Steeple sign on an x-ray indicates subglottic tracheal narrowing, which is indicative of the diagnosis of croup.
22) **Correct answer: D** Succinylcholine has been shown to cause acute rhabdomyolysis, ventricular dysrhythmias, cardiac arrest and death in apparently healthy children after administration. These children were usually subsequently found to have undiagnosed skeletal muscle myopathies.

Chapter 18 | Study Tips

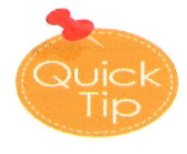

- *Study and sufficiently prepare.*
- *Take notes during the lecture and go back and review those notes.*
- *Go back and find weak areas and focus on them.*
- *Time management – be sure to know how much time can be spent on each question.*
- *If you have the ability to go back, write down questions you were unsure about and go back and look at them again instead of staying on the question too long. Limit (1) minute per question.*
- *Most of the time, these tests allow you more than enough time to finish the exam.*
- *Be sure to read the question slowly and fully to understand what is being asked of you.*
- *Beware of distractions – don't get caught up in the scenario. Read the last couple of sentences to determine what is being asked of you.*
- *Pay close attention to phrases such as: EXCEPT.*
- <u>*Eliminate the distractors and wrong answers first; this usually leaves you with two good answers; be able to select the best answer of the two.*</u>
- *Don't skip questions.*
- *Think about your answer before you look at the choices; this may help you with the correct answer or to jog your memory to determine the correct answer.*
- *There are usually trigger words in questions to make you automatically think of the answer - C/P that is stabbing and radiating into the back – think aneurysm. Referred (L) shoulder pain – think spleen.*
- *Use the paper or board supplied to you for quick numbers you want to remember.*
- *Hit problem areas right before the test and write down any numbers or values that you think might help you.*
- *Get plenty of rest and eat a good breakfast.*

References

Alspach, J. (Ed.). (1998). *Core curriculum for critical care nursing* (6th Ed.). Philadelphia, PA: Saunders Elsevier

American College of Surgeons (2012). *Advanced trauma life support student course manual* 9th Ed. Philadelphia: Lippincott, Williams & Wilkins

American Heart Association & American Academy of Pediatrics. (2000). *Neonatal resuscitation textbook* (4th Ed.). Elk Grove Village: American Academy of Pediatrics

ARDS Network. (1998). *Prospective, randomized, multi-center trial of 12 ml/kg vs. 6 ml/kg tidal volume positive pressure ventilation for treatment of acute lung injury and acute respiratory distress syndrome (ARMA)*. ARDSNet Study 01, Version III. Retrieved from http://www.ardsnet.org/system/files/armaprotocolV3_1998-09-11_0.pdf

Darovic, G. (2002). *Hemodynamic monitoring invasive and non-invasive clinical application* 3rd Ed. Philadelphia: W.B. Saunders Co

Dellinger, R., Mitchell, L. M., Rhodes, A., Annane, D., Gerlach, H., & Opal, S. M. (2013, February). Surviving sepsis campaign: international guidelines for management of severe sepsis and septic shock: 2012. *Critical Care Medicine, 41*(2), 580-636. Retrieved from www.ccmjournal.org

Guy, J. (2007, March 13). Oxygenation and PEEP. ICU Rounds Podcast. Nashville, TN, USA.
Fischbach, F. (2004). *A manual of laboratory and diagnostic tests* (7th Ed.). Philadelphia, PA: Lippincott Williams & Wilkins

Guyton, A., & Hall, J. (2000). *Textbook of medical physiology* (10th Ed.). Philadelphia, PA: W.B. Saunders Elsevier

Holleran, R. (Ed.). (2005). *Air and surface patient transport: Principles & practice* (3rd Ed.). Philadelphia, PA: Elsevier Health Sciences

Holleran, R. (Ed.). (2010). *Air and surface patient transport: Principles & practice* (4th Ed.). Philadelphia, PA: Elsevier Health Sciences

Kattwinkel J. (Ed.) (2006). Neonatal resuscitation textbook 5th Ed. Dallas: American Academy of Pediatrics & American Heart Association

Marino, P. L. (1998). *The ICU book* (2nd ed.). (S. R. Zinner, Ed.) Baltimore, MD: Lippincott Williams & Wilkins

McIntosh, L. (1997). *Essentials of nurse anesthesia*. New York: McGraw-Hill Companies Inc.

Mejia, R. (Ed.). (2008). *Pediatric fundamental critical care support*. Mount Prospect, IL: Society of Critcal Care Medicine

Neligan, P. (2006). Acute Lung Injury. Retrieved from Critical Care Medicine Tutorials:

http://www.ccm tutorials.com/rs/ali/vili.htm

Neligan, P. (2006, December). Critical Care Medicine Tutorials. Retrieved from All about Oxygen: http://www.ccm tutorials.com/index.htm

Nolan, P.J. (Ed.). (1995). *Fundamentals of college physics*. Dubuque, IA: Wm. C. Brown Communications, Inc.

Pillitteri A. (2007). *Maternal & child health nursing* (5th Ed.). Philadelphia, PA: Lippincott, Williams & Wilkins

Pollack, Andrew. (Ed.). (2010). *Critical Care Transport.* Sudbury, MA: Jones and Bartlett Publishers

Surgeons, A. A. (2011). Critical Care Transport. In A. Pollack. Jones and Bartlett Learning. Retrieved from: http://www.aic.cuhk.edu.hk/web8/prvc.htm

Tintinalli, J., Kelen, G. Stapczynski, J. (Ed.). (2004) Emergency medicine: A comprehensive study guide 6th Ed. New York: McGraw-Hill Companies Inc.

Urden, L., Stacy, K., & Lough, M. (2005). *Thelan's critical care nursing diagnosis and management* (5th Ed.). Maryland Heights, MO: Elsevier Health Sciences

Walls, R., Murphy, M., Luten, R., & Schneider, R. (2008). *The manual of emergency airway management.* (3rd Ed.). Philadelphia, PA: Lippincott Williams & Wilkin

Made in the USA
Charleston, SC
27 November 2015